# *The*
# EBOLA OUTBREAK
# in WEST AFRICA

# The
# EBOLA OUTBREAK
# in WEST AFRICA

*Why?*

Constantine N. Nana, PhD

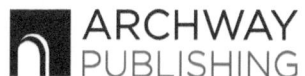

Archway Publishing books may be ordered through booksellers or by contacting:

Archway Publishing
1663 Liberty Drive
Bloomington, IN 47403
www.archwaypublishing.com
1 (888) 242-5904

ISBN: 978-1-4808-3596-2 (sc)
ISBN: 978-1-4808-3597-9 (e)

Library of Congress Control Number: 2016913735

Print information available on the last page.

Archway Publishing rev. date: 09/07/2016

*No man would keep his hands off what was not his own when he could safely take what he liked out of the market, or go into houses and lie with any one at his pleasure, or kill or release from prison whom he would, and in all respects be like a god among men*
*— Glaucon (Plato's Republic)*

*Until the lions have their own historians, the history*
*of the hunt will always favor the hunter*
*– Chinua Achebe*

# CONTENTS

# PREFACE

Since at least the 13th century, the word 'why' has been used as an adverb or conjunction to offer a suggestion as regards the cause, reason or purpose of an occurrence, or simply to express annoyance. Thus, when it is not rhetorical, the question is almost always the most difficult to answer. Where there is a chain or network of causes or reasons, the answerer is required to rank them in order of proximity or preponderance. This is a tall order where the incident in issue is an epidemic. It is even a more tedious task where the epidemic in question is the Ebola virus disease. Everything about this disease is obscure. There have been several recorded outbreaks since 1976 and in each case the lineage of the virus that caused the outbreak has simply disappeared, leaving no trace. Researchers have combed the forest on each occasion but have been unable to determine when the Ebola virus spilled over from one animal to a human. They have therefore been unable to identify the natural reservoir of the virus, and there is even no evidence that humans have disturbed this natural reservoir by hunting it for meat or dragging it out of its ecosystem. Also intriguing is that the researchers submit that the virus cannot be effectively adapted for use as a weapon of war, but yet when they apply for funding they postulate that the virus remains a potential bioterrorism threat and measures must be adopted to respond swiftly to newly emerging and man-made versions of the virus.

What is most intriguing about the outbreak in parts of West Africa in 2014 is that despite the general incertitude in the research community, the media seemed unambiguously explicit about the chain of events. They were categorical about a two-year-old child in a village in Guinea hunting bats in a hollow tree and returning home with the Ebola virus. The more I spoke with researchers, the more I realized that the accounts in the media grossly misrepresented the findings of field researchers to the point of verging on skullduggery. It is against this background that I set to answer the question most have asked, but few have attempted to answer: why? I sought to answer this question by simply establishing factual causation. In other words, use causation to connect the conduct of the reservoir (natural or artificial) with the resulting effect (the epidemic). However, I soon realized that this outbreak was even more enigmatic than the previous ones given that it was caused by the Zaire Ebola virus which normally resides about two thousand miles away. Before the outbreak, there was no indication that the Zaire Ebola virus was present in West Africa. Several conspiracy theories are offered on the Internet, and although the bulk of them are baseless, they raise some pertinent questions: why were there Ebola experts in the region shortly before the outbreak? Why did the Sierra Leonean government order a research institution to stop "Ebola testing" during the outbreak? Why did the government of the United States decline to renew funding for one of the research programs during the crisis (when the money was most needed)? Why did one of the key researchers state that the epidemic may have been caused by a contaminated needle? The more I have read about the outbreak, the more it has become evident that it is a toss-up between the Ebola virus spilling over from an unknown animal to an unknown human at an unknown location, and a human clinical trial that went wrong or accidental exposure in a laboratory.

# CHAPTER 1

# The Setting

Shortly after the outbreak of the Ebola virus disease in parts of West Africa, an epidemiologic investigation conducted by Baize et al. (published in *The New England Journal of Medicine*, 2014) confirmed the origin of the disease in the village of Meliandou. This village has since become notorious around the world and even has a page on Wikipedia. Nonetheless, there are only five lines about the village on the page. The first line describes its location in the Gueckedou Prefecture in the Nzerekore Region of southern Guinea, and the remaining four lines are about the village's connection to the Ebola virus disease. This connection is largely based on the findings of the investigation conducted by Baize et al. given that it has since been cited repeatedly by commentators and media across the world. Baize et al. collected data on possible transmission chains from hospital records and through interviews with public health authorities, patients, affected families, and neighbors. It is this data that motivated them to conclude that the Ebola virus may have left its unknown reservoir, conveyed by some mode of transmission, and infected the first susceptible human host in the village of Meliandou. However, it is interesting that no confirmed case was identified in the village, and the suspected cases had all died before the investigation even began. Thus, there was no infected person in the village at the time. It may then be contended that this was the case of following tracks on the basis of narratives and concluding with a strong presumption that the chain of infection began in Meliandou. Although there is a good reason for assuming that Meliandou is where it all began, it is also possible that no person infected with the Ebola virus ever lived in that village. The Lassa hemorrhagic fever with symptoms similar to the Ebola virus disease is endemic in the region and accounts for up to a third of deaths in hospitals there. The disease develops after an incubation period of 6 to 21 weeks. Hence, given the uncertainty as regards the date of the passing on of the alleged Patient Zero, it is possible that the latter and members of his family may have been killed by the Lassa hemorrhagic fever.

Meliandou is a forested area with an estimated population of just 719. It is nestled in beautiful verdant hills and tall, dark green trees but hosts some of the most impoverished people of the proud Republic of Guinea. The country has a population of over 10.5 million. Despite the fact that it is the second largest producer of bauxite on the planet, and has large deposits of diamonds and gold, it is a poverty mill like most of its African counterparts. Thus, in order to vary the cadence, the deadly Ebola virus disease was added to the mix. The question 'why' remains unanswered and it may be the case for the next century given that the previous outbreaks in Sudan, Zaire (the former name of the Democratic Republic of Congo), Uganda, and Gabon remain an enigma even to the most assiduous of researchers. The findings of the study by Baize et al. nonetheless spurred many on to believing that answers may be buried in Meliandou. Hence, since the outbreak, many have journeyed or gone on an expedition to the hamlet. It is a two days' drive from the capital city of Conakry, jouncing as you ride on the bumpy and dense clay path right into the heart of darkness;

as Joseph Conrad envisaged Africa forever to be. Vehicles cannot go into the hamlet itself, and so the inquisitive travelers are required to continue afoot through the leafy rainforest. They are welcomed by bright white smiles and makeshift huts made of wooden logs and thatched roofs, as well as old and frowzy concrete buildings with discolored aluminum sheets on the roofs.

However, it is not an immersion or experiential trip. The visitors do not care for the local culture and would not sample the local cuisine to save their lives. They are erudite and have read many articles about the local populace eating bats, and that the latter is the likely reservoir or the long-term host of the Ebola virus. The habitat in which this very dreaded virus thrives and multiplies. As noted above, Meliandou is notorious for being the scene of transmission; where Patient Zero allegedly accosted the sole mysterious bat hosting the Ebola virus and enabled the pathogen to be transmitted from its long-term host to susceptible humankind. So the visitors tread lightly around the hut in which the alleged Patient Zero lived. With pompous reverence, they talk to the generous but ever-so-addled father of the alleged Patient Zero, who speaks of his unease at being a rather macabre attraction. The visitors are also keen to see the hollow tree in which Patient Zero allegedly encountered the infected insectivorous free-tailed bat, about fifty meters from the family home. However, they are treated only to a stump clogged with soot. The story is that the hollow tree was consumed by fire sometime in the middle of March 2014. The fire killed several bats, including most likely the mysterious free-tailed bat that had infected the alleged Patient Zero.

I must admit that the slightly cynical tone adopted in describing the above events is motivated by profound skepticism about Meliandou being where it all began. As will be shown below, this does not imply that I endorse conspiracy theories about the causes of the Ebola virus disease outbreak in parts of West Africa. George Santayana said:

"profound skepticism is favorable to conventions, because it doubts that the criticism of conventions is any truer than they are." Thus, in spite of the strong expression of disapproval of the accepted chain of infection and probable cause of the Ebola virus disease outbreak, the conclusion that is drawn here is that the postulate of the Ebola virus leaving its unknown reservoir and infecting the first susceptible human host in the village of Meliandou, seems as undependable as criticisms of the postulate. Given that I believe the postulate of the virus infecting a child in Meliandou awaits demonstration, I shall cease discussing the village at this point. After analyzing several journal articles, books, reports in newspapers, and opinion pieces, I am more inclined to surmise that Ground Zero was in the Republic of Sierra Leone (Kenema) and not Meliandou in neighboring Guinea.

Subsequent studies have shown that there are possible Ebola antibodies in human blood samples that were drawn from some patients in Sierra Leone long before the Ebola virus disease outbreak in 2013 and 2014. As such, humans in that country may have come into contact with the Ebola virus well before the first confirmed cases in March 2014 and suspected cases in December 2013. Other studies have revealed that some people in this country may have an immune response to the virus given that they have never presented with symptoms after sustained exposure to the virus. The questions that remain unanswered are how did the patients with Ebola antibodies come into contact with the virus; and what was the transmission mechanism? The thorough search for answers in Meliandou has been futile because they may be buried in Kenema after all.

## KENEMA

There are four principal administrative divisions in the Republic of Sierra Leone, namely the Western Area, Northern Province, Southern Province, and Eastern Province. The Eastern Province has a picturesque countryside with spectacular views of the Gola Hills and Loma Mountains, the most prominent massifs of two range systems. The topography of the region is sufficient reason for tourists to flock to the Eastern Province each year, but alas, the promotion of tourist travel for commercial purposes is seldom a top priority of African governments. Despite the fact that these governments lord over an awe-inspiring topography and could potentially offer what no other continent on the planet can, tourism is deemed to be anecdotal; a perfunctory effort to please curious European rovers and ambitious researchers. Granted, international travel for short leisure breaks is not a common habit of Africans, and most tourism policies are geared toward setting up small-scale projects in local communities to enable tourists' money reach the hinterlands (pro-poor tourism). But then again, it is uncertain why a lot of resources are not allocated to cultural tourism, promoting the invaluable heritage of the area. Logically, the poor state of tourism may be due to the fact that there is no decent infrastructure (youth hostels, halls, auditoriums, etc.) to cater for tourists, especially the low budget travelers. In fact, saying that there is no decent infrastructure is Afrocentric euphemism. For an industry that employs about eight thousand Sierra Leoneans, the gateway to this touristic idyll is the dysfunctional and shabby Freetown-Lungi International Airport.

Notwithstanding, the Sierra Leonean Ministry of Tourism describes the country as "Africa's Hidden Paradise" – it is anyone's guess why this "paradise" remains hidden. Given the government's inability to effectively highlight the country's rich heritage, its stigmatization by foreign media as a hotbed of Ebola has now turned some of its most picturesque areas into a "dark site" for dark tourism. Thus, it may only attract researchers, journalists, and the tourists with macabre curiosity seeking to observe the devastation caused by the cruel disease. One of such "dark sites" is no doubt the Eastern Province. Dark tourists are attracted not by the Gola Hills and Loma Mountains but by the infamy of Kenema.

Kenema is an ethnically diverse town of just under two hundred thousand people in the Eastern Province. As the third largest conglomerate in the country, it comprises six municipalities. However, the general management of the town is the responsibility of a mayor, the executive head of an elected council. The Eastern Province shares borders with six different administrative divisions, three of which belong to the State of Liberia and one to the Republic of Guinea. Amongst the six divisions is Nzerekore in Guinea, the division in which Meliandou is located. Thus, given that Kenema is the main urban center in the six divisions, as well as of the entire Eastern Province, it is only natural that it is burdened with the task of resolving the problems that overwhelm the few institutions in these largely rural divisions. One of such problems is health care. Health administration is a prominent and unswerving headache in all six divisions, as well as the rest of the Eastern Province, as well as the rest of Sierra Leone, as well as the rest of Africa. In fact, it is as prominent as the fecklessness of the respective governments in directing their efforts toward what is clearly the most salient plight of the people. As noted above, the highly contagious acute viral hemorrhagic fever known as Lassa fever is regularly found among people in these divisions. The multimammate rodent (*Mastomys natalensis*) that spread the Lassa virus to humans live in a cross-section of households and are often eaten in some areas. Efforts at ensuring that the largely indigent and unwitting inhabitants maintain effective personal hygiene, and also that the rodents are kept away from cooking pots and dark corners of houses have for the most part been futile. There are still roughly between 300,000 and 500,000 cases of Lassa fever each year, causing about 5,000 fatalities.

It may be contended that Sierra Leone epitomizes the paradox of poverty in modern Africa. It is among the top fifteen diamond producing countries on the planet with annual production estimated at US$300 million. It has one of the largest deposits of rutile. This is a mineral that contains titanium dioxide, iron, niobium, and tantalum; and is used for the manufacture of refractory ceramic. It is also used as a pigment in paints, plastics, paper, and various applications that require a bright white color. The mining of rutile near the village of Bonthe in Sierra Leone began in 1979. By 1990, it was the largest non-petroleum investment of the United States in West Africa, with export earnings of approximately US$75 million. Although the operations were suspended after rebels took over the mining site in 1995, they resumed some ten years later.

Despite these natural resources, Sierra Leone boasts of one of the worst public health systems around the world. It may conveniently be ranked among the worst fifteen public health systems on the planet – although ranking the public health systems of West African countries in the order of inadequacy is like grading the different oceans according to wetness. It is uncertain why health care is not the Sierra Leonean government's top strategic priority. Programs such as the Free Health Care Initiative that provide medical treatment to pregnant women free of charge are commendable. However, they should not be outside of the normal expectations of citizens. One of the major producers of gem-quality diamonds on the planet should at the very least be able to provide decent health care to its 6.1 million citizens. Blame may also be assigned to foreign smugglers of contraband weapons, as well as traders in 'blood diamond' or the donor countries and institutions. Nonetheless, every reasonable and objective observer would establish a link between the acute corruption of officials and the government's failure or negligence in managing the exploitation and exportation of the minerals. This is substantiated by the fact that a United Nations-approved certification system for exporting diamonds from Sierra Leone set up in October 2000 dramatically increased the volume of legal exports and money received by the treasury. In 1999, the formal exports were just US$1.9 million, but by 2001, they had increased to US$26 million, and US$142 million in 2005.

Another commendable effort (commendable efforts here are like the silver lining of John Milton's sable cloud) is the Diamond Area Community Development Fund (DACDF) that was set up by the Sierra Leonean central government in 2001 to enhance citizen participation in decision making as regards the management of mineral resources. The main objective was to increase the stake of local communities in the legal trade of the resources. Modeled on other ineffectual initiatives such as Zimbabwe's CAMPFIRE and Mali's *Gestion des Terroirs*, it was introduced with the laudable social goals of allocating more resources to the needs of indigent and vulnerable communities affected by mining operations, and enhancing the transparency and fairness of decisions about the management of the resources. Hence, a proportion of the revenue generated from the trade ought to have been returned to the communities on a consistent basis. Roy Maconachie in a chapter in a book edited by Paivi Lujala and Siri Rustad (*High-value Natural Resources: A Blessing or a Curse for Peace?*) states that the DACDF has provided a strong incentive to miners and the host communities to engage in and promote legal mining. This has, in turn, strengthened the Kimberley Process Certification Scheme for rough diamonds. This scheme is geared toward curbing the flow of 'conflict diamonds' or diamonds used to fund military operations by factions or forces opposed to legitimate and internationally recognized governments. It involves sealing the rough diamonds in tamper-resistant containers and issuing a certificate of origin with unique serial numbers each time the diamonds are transported across a national frontier. Hence, the conflict diamonds are ring-fenced to prevent their entry into the international market. All countries that refuse to endorse the international certification scheme are not allowed to trade on the international market. Most producing countries have also endorsed the World Diamond Council's proposal to ensure that invoices are accompanied by a written guarantee that the "diamonds have been purchased from legitimate sources not involved in funding conflict and in compliance with United Nations resolutions."

Laudable though the efforts and objectives might be, it is uncertain why it is the governments of exporting and importing countries that are tasked with checking all Kimberley Process certificates, given that endemic corruption and racketeering by government officers in most of these countries is common knowledge. That is as good as appointing the getaway driver warden of a penitentiary. Where government control is ineffective, it is expected that mining companies and associations would volunteer to monitor their adherence to the standards set in Kimberley, as well as enforce these standards. Thus, a half-baked self-regulation model serves as the backup plan. In 2003, Business Day described the process as a "toothless watchdog, chained to a kennel." However, by the time that article was published, the revenues from the export of diamonds had reached US$23.8 million, compared to just over US$21 million for the whole of 2002. Nonetheless, it is uncertain whether there was a direct link between the sharp rise in export earnings and the implementation of the Kimberley Process. By 2001, the clout of the Revolutionary United Front (RUF), the rebel army that sought to topple the Sierra Leonean government, had been lessened so much so that the rebel army had been converted into a political party, the Revolutionary United Front Party. This is because the RUF had repeatedly been battered by British, Guinean, and Indian Special Forces, and its leader, Foday Sankoh, had been captured.

As such, the Kimberley Process did not break the RUF's stranglehold on the diamond trade. The British, Guinean, and Indian forces did. Notwithstanding, the then Sierra Leonean Mineral Resources Minister, Mohamed Swarray-Deen, was full of praise of the Kimberley Process in an article published on the website of the *Agence France-Presse* in 2003. He noted that it had "returned the diamond industry back to the community which is rightly the main beneficiary." He also intimated that the Process "was originally hijacked by a few greedy and corrupt people." It may then be understood that the production and trade are now transparent, and the Kimberley Process may effectively rely upon the government's vigilance. However, the irony here is obvious. The phrase "a few greedy and corrupt people" used by the Sierra Leonean Minister is often a very apt description of most African governments. Hence, what happened, in fact, is that the control of the diamond trade was taken from one small group of "greedy and corrupt people" and handed over to another small group of greedy and corrupt people; much like what happened during the 'independence' of many African countries. Notwithstanding, at the time Mohamed Swarray-Deen made that statement, a Lebanese merchant was cited by the *Agence France-Presse* as intimating that "other individual powerful interests have stepped in to keep both illicit mining and smuggling alive. They have their contacts in Conakry and Monrovia ... There are lots of mafia-like movements involved."

It may nonetheless be argued that what is important is that export earnings have increased sharply since the end of the civil war and the inception of the Kimberley Process. However, there has been no proportional increase in investment in healthcare and sanitation. As deplored above, it is uncertain why health care is not the government's top strategic priority. It is indeed bewildering that a country with so many health problems should spend so little (relatively) on health care and sanitation. It seems that as earnings have increased the budget allocations to the health sector, as well as the disbursements have reduced.

A study conducted by the Budget Advocacy Network showed that the Sierra Leonean government pursued the 'policy' of waiting for the disease to strike. It may not be presumptuous to contend that the same policy was effectively in place prior to the outbreak of the Ebola virus disease in 2014. The report of the Budget Advocacy Network showed that although the health budget increased by 4.9% between 2007 and 2011, it dropped by 17.5% in 2012. This seriously compromised the government's ability to sustain the Free Health Care Initiative. The good news is that the actual annual expenditure for health care increased at an average rate of 59.3% between 2007 and 2012. It even surpassed the budgeted allocation in 2012. But then again, some vital program areas including maternal and child health, school health, malaria prevention and control, and STI/HIV/AIDS prevention and control experienced substantial funding cuts from the allocated budget of 2010. The Budget Advocacy Network logically deplored these cuts on the grounds that they would negatively impact on primary, secondary, and tertiary health care given that many institutions were left unable to provide basic care or run preventive programs. Also, the actual stock of drugs for treating diarrhea, malaria, fever, and measles was absent. Given the high incidence of disease in Sierra Leone, it is astonishing that the government is impudent enough to impose any cuts. The citizens of the country seem to continue to rely heavily on private or non-governmental initiatives. One of the most laudable of such initiatives is the Kenema Government Hospital.

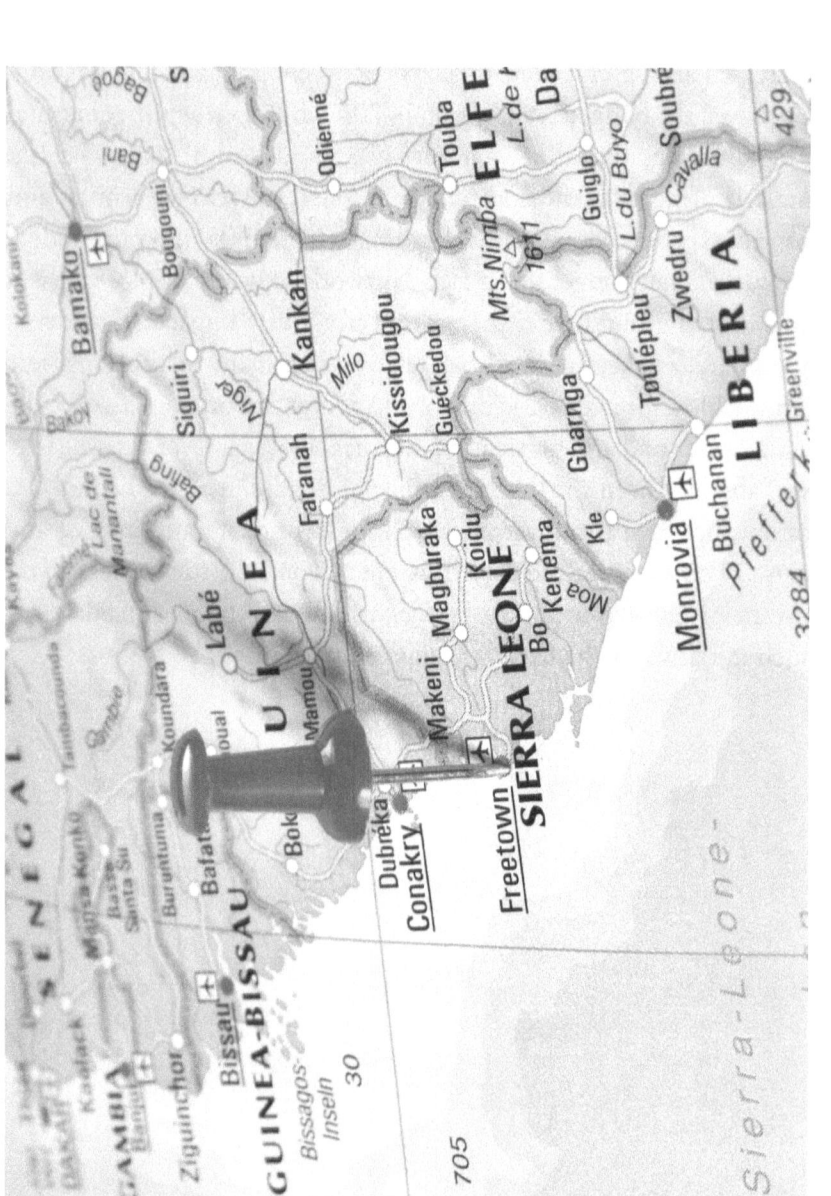

*Political Map of West Africa (the southern part affected by the epidemic).*

## THE KENEMA GOVERNMENT HOSPITAL

This healthcare institution was built in Kenema thanks to the World Health Organization (WHO) and the United Nations Mission in Sierra Leone (UNAMSIL). The International Committee of the Red Cross (ICRC) also helped in furnishing the institution with the donation of surgical supplies, plastic sheeting, blankets, and drugs for the treatment of the war-wounded during the civil war. Working with the patients of the hospital facilitated the implementation of the ICRC's Tracing Program for missing persons. Other organizations that have been of immense help include the Medical Emergency Relief International (MERLIN) that donated nutritional feeding to the poorly nourished in a malnutrition center that was specially established in the hospital. The glaring absence of African institutions and businesses on the list of sponsors is unsurprising. Nonetheless, the hospital has many well-equipped laboratories to facilitate the rapid diagnoses of the myriad of diseases affecting the area. HIV prevalence was 1.9% in 2005, and the Kenema Government Hospital was the only HIV testing site in the District. The incidence of Lassa fever, Yellow fever, Tuberculosis, and Malaria in the area are also relatively very high. The incidence of Lassa fever was particularly high and prompted the expansion of the hospital with the creation of the Lassa Fever Ward. This is a biomedical unit that was devoted to both patient care and research on viral hemorrhagic fevers. Between 2005 and 2014, the unit was managed by Sheikh Umar Khan, who later on played a prominent role in the perilous and treacherous fight against the Ebola virus disease in Sierra Leone. Chapter 6 discusses his role and very tragic demise.

The administrators, healthcare personnel, and researchers took great pride in the Lassa Fever Ward. In 2005, an article by Mohammed Massaquoi on the website of the Africa News Service announced that a "first class Lassa Fever Laboratory" had been handed over

to the Kenema Government Hospital by the Special Representative
of the Secretary-General of UNAMSIL, the late Daudi Mwakago.
Massaquoi also mentioned that the ceremony was grand and well
attended, and the enchanted crowd was told that this was part of
UNAMSIL's commitment to the development of Sierra Leone. The
crowd was also informed that the laboratory would be oriented toward
applied research in communicable diseases.

Two years later, Alyson Zureick of the International Rescue Committee
(IRC) visited the maternity ward of the Hospital. This ward had just
received essential drugs and supplies, as well as technical assistance
from the IRC. On a blog on Skoll World Forum, she gave a more
somber description of the institution which she described as "a prime
example of how the government is struggling to provide essential
services to the population." She noted that the hospital is located off
a dusty roadway, and several portions of the road material had broken
away leaving many potholes. The hospital's sinuous open air corridors
and small wards were poignant features that she remembered quite
well. Ambulances provided by the IRC and managed by a group of
local drivers were regularly used. One of the ambulances brought a
young pregnant woman suffering from obstructed labor who later
on gave birth to a baby girl through C-section. Alyson Zureick
noted that obstructed labor or labor dystocia was among the most
preventable causes of maternal and perinatal mortality in the region.
She also intimated that poor access to medical care during labor and
pregnancy was a major cause of maternal death, and Sierra Leone had
one of the highest rates on the planet. Nonetheless, the introduction
of ambulances had helped in saving the pregnancies and lives of many
young women and infants. Like most visitors, she noticed that the
hospital was unable to meet up with the surge in health care demand
in the entire region. Also, there were often shortages of essential drugs
and other supplies. This was compounded by inadequate staffing in
the various wards. During her visit, she was told that the maternity

ward had a single obstetrician-gynecologist and just three doctors on call. This was only logical since there were only about 200 fully trained physicians in the entire country, and many preferred to live and work in private clinics in the capital city, Freetown. Also, there was no social security. Hence, apart from the ruling elite, only a few lucky patients with insufficient or no income received monetary assistance from international agencies and local NGOs.

The Lassa Fever Ward comprised two sections. The first section was used for routine diagnostics, and the second section was a Biosafety Level 2 laboratory. Thus, the latter section was used for work that involved pathogens of moderate potential hazard such as viruses and bacteria that caused only mild disease to humans or which were difficult to contract via aerosol. Understandably, access to the Biosafety Level 2 section was limited, and the members of staff that were allowed into the laboratory had specific training in handling the pathogens. Also, it may be assumed that extreme precautions were taken when working in the section. There is nothing to suggest that the staff were not sufficiently cautious or that the Director of the Laboratory and the three technicians did not exercise the proper standard of care at all times. However, a quick glance at the picture of the laboratory on the Viral Hemorrhagic Fever Consortium's website revealed how impetuous it was to set up a Biosafety Level 2 laboratory in a ruinous shack that looked more like one of those mangy taverns in the abandoned backcountry that was visited only by lighthearted and devil-may-care loafers. That would only be reasonable if the laboratory were an underground unit like Dr. Kananga's subterranean lair of operations. Perhaps the problem was that all medication (that is the very limited stock) at the ward was provided free of charge by the government. Nevertheless, no one would be frightened out of their wits by the harum-scarum ways of African governments and health authorities. But then again, it is a bit of a stretch to allow samples from suspected Lassa fever cases to be handled in such a dingy cabin.

Notwithstanding, it was noted on the website of the Consortium that this was the only Lassa Isolation Unit in the world. As flattering as this may sound, one wonders why several world-renowned research institutions and experts (see next Chapter) who received awards of huge sums of money would choose to work in such a ruinous building rather than allocate part of their grants to building a state-of-the-art facility.

Despite the shoddiness of the Lassa Fever Ward, only the bumptious commentator would disparage the facility outright. It was not only better than anything ever offered by the Sierra Leonean government, but it is important to note that it was there thanks to the charity of foreigners. It may still be difficult to argue in some quarters that such structures are erected on the basis of pure benevolence given the history of surreptitious human clinical trials in Africa. However, until evidence is adduced to that effect, such a feeling betrays presumptuous ingratitude. Notwithstanding, it is surprising that the government of the United States decided in August 2014 not to renew funding for the project on Lassa fever and thereby cut resources that were channeled to patient care and research at the Lassa Fever Ward. What is most intriguing is that this decision was taken at a time when this unit had more or less become the 'Ebola ward', given that it was used to treat the large numbers of patients who had contracted the lethal Ebola virus disease. A contracting officer for the National Institute of Allergy and Infectious Diseases of the National Institutes of Health (NIH) intimated that the proposal for the renewal of funding submitted by Tulane University had been rejected "based on technical factors, scientific priority, and availability of funds." The NIH declined to provide any clarifications or even comment further. The timing of the decision and the uncertainty as regards the NIH's motivation certainly raise many questions: was the decision related to the US government's decision to cut spending? Does the uncommunicative posture imply the NIH had caught a whiff of something unethical cooking in Kenema prior to the outbreak of the Ebola virus disease?

The NIH's reticence, the ambivalence of the theory about the source of the Ebola virus, the fictitious narrative about a two-year-old boy encountering an infected free-tailed bat in a hollow tree, and the general uncertainty about the reservoir of the virus in previous outbreaks all meld into a presentiment of conspiracy. The presentiment inspires questions such as that about something unethical being carried out in the Lassa Fever Ward prior to the outbreak. It may also inspire conspiracy theories such as the many theories offered on the Internet on the arcane causes of the outbreak. It may also inspire a questioning attitude toward opinions and unempirical knowledge which were presented as established facts and the official narrative. That is the attitude I invariably adopted in analyzing the facts on the outbreak.

## THE OUTBREAK

The Viral Hemorrhagic Fever Consortium was satisfied that the staff at the Lassa Fever Ward adhered to strict universal precautions when dealing with patients. This vote of confidence was seriously tested at the outbreak of the Ebola virus disease in mid-2014. On the website of the WHO, it was noted that the first *confirmed* case in Kenema and Sierra Leone was a young woman who turned up with a high fever and was bleeding profusely following a miscarriage. This was on May 24, 2014, more than two months after the first confirmed (not suspected) cases in neighboring Guinea. As such, a health worker at the Kenema Government Hospital suspected the young woman could be suffering from the Ebola virus disease since there were reports of an outbreak in the Gueckedou Prefecture in the Nzerekore Region of southern Guinea. As noted above, Kenema is the main urban center in the six neighboring divisions (including Nzerekore) and is burdened with the task of resolving the problems that overwhelm the few institutions in these largely rural divisions. It is therefore only natural that the Kenema Government Hospital received the most difficult cases in the region. However, it is surprising that it received its first Ebola case more than two months after the first confirmed cases in Nzerekore. Amongst the earliest victims was a healthcare worker who instead went to the less equipped Macenta Hospital in Gueckedou rather than the Kenema Government Hospital that had a better stock of drugs for treating diarrhea and hemorrhagic fever, as well as an isolation ward. Moreover, there were many hemorrhagic fever experts from around the world working at or with the Lassa Fever Ward of the Kenema Government Hospital. That notwithstanding, it is sometimes difficult to rationalize the decisions made by patients, especially when in the throes of a lethal disease such as the Ebola virus disease.

The young woman who checked into the Kenema Government Hospital on May 24, 2014, was tested for Ebola and placed in isolation the next day. The test confirmed the fears of the personnel, and they immediately notified the Sierra Leonean Ministry of Health and Sanitation, which in turn notified the WHO about the occurrence of the Ebola virus disease in Sierra Leone. However, this should not have been unexpected in light of the outbreak a few months earlier in the neighboring villages in Guinea. Moreover, the Kenema Government Hospital was the reference hospital for hemorrhagic fever not only in the affected villages but countries. This explains why all the requisite precautions were taken with the first reported case of Ebola at this hospital. The young patient recovered fully in the isolation ward, and no patient or member of the staff was infected. Maybe the efficiency and competence demonstrated in this case made the medical staff overconfident about their ability to manage an outbreak in Kenema. They allegedly tracked the source of the young patient's infection to the burial of a revered traditional healer. It seemed they then found out that the traditional healer's shrine was a more celebrated healing institution than the Kenema Government Hospital. Patients suffering from hemorrhagic fever (the patients did not know it was the Ebola virus disease) had allegedly been taken by their families to the traditional healer's shrine rather than the Kenema Government Hospital. It cannot be said that the decision was motivated by the cost of the treatment since all medication at the Lassa Fever Ward was provided free of charge by the government. Thus, given that Lassa fever is a hemorrhagic fever, it is intriguing that a patient suffering from a hemorrhagic fever would not immediately think of the institution of reference, where medication is provided free of charge. However, as noted above, it is sometimes difficult to rationalize the decisions made by patients, especially when in the throes of a lethal disease such as the Ebola virus disease. It is alleged that the traditional healer contracted the disease from one of his many patients and died. The virus was then ironically transmitted to mourners who came to pay their last respects, and then spread across several villages. The principle is that disease can spread quickly in healthcare settings, although in this instance, the setting was the shrine of a traditional healer.

Nonetheless, by the middle of June 2014, patients were flocking to the Kenema Government Hospital, may be prompted by the story of the young woman who had been cured of the Ebola virus disease, or may be due to the fact that smaller clinics in the neighboring villages were overwhelmed, or may be due to the fact that traditional healers had themselves become an endangered species. Thus, it was only a matter of time before the Kenema Government Hospital was equally swept away by the deluge. In an article published in *The New York Times* on September 12, 2014, Pardis Sabeti states that the then Director of the Lassa Fever War, Sheikh Umar Khan, and other personnel isolated the first reported case and used personal protective equipment (PPE) while treating her until she made a full recovery. Hence, isolation preventive measures were properly implemented, and the virus was not transmitted to any other person. She also notes that the personnel of the hospital was fully aware of the likelihood of being infected by the Ebola virus in the near future given that the outreach team had discovered that at least 14 people were infected in the patient's village, and the disease was spreading exponentially. As such, the subsequent infection of several healthcare workers at the Kenema Government Hospital was not a case of the medical staff confusing Ebola fever patients for Lassa fever patients. Pardis Sabeti seems to give the impression that the situation got out of hand while Sheikh Umar Khan was attending the inauguration of the African Center of Excellence for Genomics of Infectious Diseases in Nigeria. She said on his return from Nigeria, the hospital was overwhelmed as the health personnel had to treat over 80 patients at a time and work for 16 hours a day. Hence, the influx of infected patients into the hospital made it impossible for the health personnel to implement isolation preventive measures effectively; in a matter of months, over 40 healthcare workers had been infected.

This implies that the health personnel knew what to do as regards prevention and sought to implement the appropriate measures, but they were soon overwhelmed as they had no meaningful external help. No organization with sufficient resources was there to coordinate activities and ensure that viable diagnostic facilities could be set up in other medical centers to test, isolate and treat infected persons. This further implies that neither the government of Sierra Leone nor the WHO saw the outbreak as an emergency requiring immediate action. They had been informed in May of 2014 of the first confirmed case in Sierra Leone. So two months later, they watched the fledgling Kenema Government Hospital drown in the deluge of Ebola patients and could not mobilize the requisite resources to assist the overwhelmed healthcare workers. In an article by Kemo Cham published in *Africa Review* (July 22, 2014), the Sierra Leonean Minister of Health and Sanitation, Miatta Kargbo, is cited as denying reports of the shortage of PPE for healthcare workers. There were reports of a strike by healthcare workers in affected areas, and church Ministers expressed frustration with the government's reluctance to declare a state of national emergency.

It is not surprising that the surviving healthcare workers went on strike following the death of their colleagues from the Ebola virus disease. The workers claimed the Sierra Leonean Ministry of Health and Sanitation had bungled every attempt to manage the epidemic and failed to give them commensurate remuneration. They also asked for the Lassa Fever Ward (that had become the 'Ebola ward') to be relocated from within the hospital, and for management responsibilities to be transferred to the international non-governmental organization, *Médecins Sans Frontières*. However, one wonders if the workers would have requested for the latter if they knew their leader, Sheikh Umar Khan, had died slowly and painfully at the hands of *Médecins Sans Frontières*, while its experts dithered about whether to administer clinically tested experimental drugs to the physician. Nonetheless, it is important to reiterate that the Sierra Leonean government's incompetence was abysmal.

In an article published on the website of the Sierra Leonean *News Watch* (December 04, 2014), it is stated that the healthcare workers had not been paid risk allowances for eight weeks, and they did not only go on strike but also "traded with" and "littered dead bodies." It is uncertain what the latter entails. Notwithstanding, this article also revealed the state of mind of the average Sierra Leonean during the crisis. Many readers would be surprised to note that it was not that of an alarmed individual. It seems while the rest of the world was panicky and hysterical, the epicenter was impassive and almost incautious. The article noted that news of the outbreak of the disease in the country was greeted with skepticism by people who thought the news was politically motivated. The fact that the most affected area was Kailahun, an opposition stronghold, was interpreted as the government's ploy to reduce the number of people voting for the main opposition party. Then the President of the Republic seemed to be engaging himself in more fruitful investments of his energy when the news of the outbreak broke. The Ebola virus is a lethal pathogen that could potentially wipe out a good chunk of a country's population. Hence, the President's tardy response and statement to the nation was almost disrespectful. He subsequently appealed to the members of his cabinet and other officials involved in managing the crisis to stop embezzling funds allocated to this cause as that was "blood money." For the President to make such a statement, prosecutions, convictions, and hefty sentences ought to have ensued, but alas, it was a fustian speech.

A report by the Auditor-General published on February 13, 2015, revealed that 30 percent of the US$19 million allegedly spent by the Sierra Leonean government in managing the crisis had been disbursed without proper supporting documentation. It stated that the Ministry of Health and Sanitation had issued poorly written contracts and failed to carry out due diligence on the winners of bids. Also, there was no evidence that incentive payments had been made to frontline healthcare workers. There were "ghost names" on some lists of healthcare workers, and the Ministry could not account for some payments. It is interesting that the Office of the President of the Republic submitted the Auditor-General's report to Parliament rather than the police.

Also, the Chief Executive Office of the National Ebola Response Center, Major Paolo Conteh, was imperious and haughty in dealing with the striking healthcare workers. He said their industrial action was politically motivated. *News Watch* reported that some of the workers were summarily dismissed. The Sierra Leone *Telegraph* published an article on February 14, 2015, entitled "Massive Misappropriation of Ebola Funds Uncovered in Sierra Leone," in which it stated that the funds allocated to the fight against the Ebola virus disease were held in a bank account managed by Major Paolo Conteh and the Minister of Health and Sanitation, Abu Bakarr Fofanah. It noted that the State House and Office of the First Lady had not accounted for over US$5 million that was transferred to their coffers. It also noted that members of the current government had "siphoned off" about US$200 million. It then concluded with the sad reminder that 12 physicians and over 200 healthcare professionals had died since the outbreak of the Ebola virus disease due to the lack of adequate protective gear. It also added a Rabelaisian note that there is "widespread suspicion that the State House and several key ruling party executives do not seriously want to see the end of Ebola in Sierra Leone – at least not before the end of 2015, by which time it would be too late to make preparations for the 2017 elections."

Nonetheless, by July 2015, there were more confirmed cases in Sierra Leone than in Guinea. According to the WHO, Sierra Leone had 336 confirmed cases, while Guinea had 301. Also, Liberia had 196. Despite the shortcomings of the Sierra Leonean authorities, there is nothing to suggest that the Guinean health authorities, largely directed and guided by the WHO and *Médecins Sans Frontières*, had adopted a particularly estimable approach (that did not promote embezzlement and mismanagement) when compared with that of their Sierra Leonean counterparts. Granted, President Alpha Conde of Guinea adopted a more hands-on approach and declared a national health emergency in March 2014. However, what is most intriguing is the lack of interest in both countries in identifying the source of the outbreak and determining how the Zaire Ebola virus appeared out of thin air and killed thousands of their people. What if the outbreak was caused by a bungled human clinical trial or an ambitious researcher's exposure to a frozen sample that had been sneaked into the region? The vast majority of studies on the epidemiology and changes in the RNA of the Ebola virus are published by American, European, and Asian researchers. The Sierra Leonean and Guinean (West African) researchers that ought to have a much better understanding of the local culture and habits of the affected people are as scarce as the bones of antediluvian animals. It is true that the Western media (Western Europe and the United States) are only keen on hearing from West African patients and families of patients, but it also seems that West African governments are just as dismissive of their researchers. For example, very little is known of Sheikh Umar Khan's ideas and the research that he was conducting together with six other Sierra Leonean healthcare workers shortly before they all suddenly died. Everything about the physician and his ideas is found in articles published by European and American researchers. Apart from banners carrying his name and face, there is nothing to suggest that the Sierra Leoneans take much interest in the man. When members of government are more interested in kickbacks from companies that win bids for building low-rent facilities with Ebola funds, it is not surprising that identifying the source of the outbreak should be the least of their priorities.

# CHAPTER 2

# The Viral Hemorrhagic Fever Consortium (The Consortium)

Information about the outbreak of the Ebola virus disease in West Africa was received with mixed feelings in different parts of the world. For many in Europe, Asia, and North America, it was the obvious and hackneyed sarcastic retort about those Africans who have infected themselves by eating monkeys and bats. For many in Africa and poor parts of Asia, it was the obvious and overdone glorification of the state of being a victim: the result of another illegal medical experimentation by those White people. However, the possession of the latter outlook arises not only from imagined victimization but also from previous instances of illegal medical experimentation on Africans. The experience of victimization may have influenced the spread of fear in the affected African community. It is only natural that several members of this community may develop an anxiety disorder after exposure to such traumatic events. On the other hand, the fundamental attribution error or correspondence bias may explain the thwarted outlook of many non-Africans in more affluent societies. There is a disposition to focus on dispositional or personality-based explanations for the observed behavior of Africans while overlooking situational explanations. For example, if a cross-section of Africans develops an outlook that arises from the victimization of a small number of Africans, the European or American observer might consider the cross-section of Africans to be overreacting. This is a dispositional explanation. However, where a small number of Europeans or Americans are victimized, and a cross-section develops an anxiety disorder, such as following the terrorist attacks on September 11, 2001, the European or American observer would be more likely to blame the fiendish source of the aggression (radical Islam); rather than argue that the majority of Europeans or Americans are overreacting. This is a situational explanation. Hence, there is a fine line between victim blaming and delineating inappropriate post-assault behavior.

That notwithstanding, there is a small number of Europeans and Americans who, although not part of the community that was previously targeted, are inhabited with a strong feeling of foreboding. An appropriate description of them would be 'skeptics' because of their disposition to incredulity toward official explanations. They rationally recommend intellectual caution or 'suspending belief' at least until the reliability of the official explanation has been independently tested. However, they are now generally referred to as conspiracy theorists. The coinage is opportune for governments in this day and age since the term has acquired a derogatory meaning in order to dismiss the claims of the theorists easily. The term 'conspiracy theorists' is nonetheless appropriate, in spite of its derogatory connotation, where the theorists are skeptical about the official explanation because they believe the relevant event was the result of a conspiracy between influential covert organizations. In this light, since the outbreak of the Ebola virus disease in parts of West Africa, many of these theorists have pointed an accusatory finger at The Consortium for being one of the leading covert plotters.

BLOGGERS' PROFILE

Many blogs set up by 'conspiracy theorists' give the impression that The Consortium is a global criminal syndicate in the mold of Ernst Starvo Blofeld's Spectre. However, rather than build training bases for terrorists and holding the world to ransom, The Consortium allegedly builds bioweapons laboratories around the world wherein it conducts research on behalf of the United States Army Medical Research Institute of Infectious Diseases (USAMRIID). On these blogs, it is claimed that the Ebola virus disease outbreak was orchestrated by The Consortium in cahoots with the USAMRIID. It is also alleged that the kits used by the health personnel and research staff at the Kenema Government Hospital (provided by The Consortium) were either false or faked. Among the most perceptive accounts is the narrative on Winter Watch by Russ Winter, which is to the effect that The Consortium was paid US$140 million by the Department of Defense of the United States and a pharmaceutical company and leading developer of RNA therapeutics, Tekmira, to test an Ebola vaccine on humans. It provides a link to a press release on *Globe Newswire* of January 14, 2014, which states as follows: "Tekmira Doses First Subject in Human Clinical Trial of TKM-Ebola." This was about a month after the Ebola virus was mysteriously introduced into the human population in Guinea. In Tekmira's press release, Mark J. Murray, the President and CEO, noted that following compelling preclinical results they had dosed the first subject in a Phase I human clinical trial of TKM-Ebola. The latter is an anti-Ebola viral therapeutic developed by Tekmira that targets the protein in the Ebola virus. Clinical trials are conducted in a sequence of phases or steps, with each phase designed to provide answers to a research question. Phase I of the trial generally involves testing the new therapeutic or drug on a small group of humans for the first time in order to ascertain a safe dosage range and identify side effects. The researchers may be able to tell whether a new drug is safe after

Phase I in order to administer the drug to larger groups of humans in Phases II and III.

Russ Winter raises a pertinent question regarding the trial: where were the healthy volunteers recruited? However, he follows up with wild accusations. The latter often proves to be the heels of Achilles of 'conspiracy theorists.' Despite the predictive ability of the hypotheses they formulate, the fact that they then burden the hypotheses with so many assumptions makes it quite easy for critics to slash (or falsify) their claims with Occam's razor. This is a problem-solving principle put forward by an English Franciscan friar in the 14$^{th}$ century. It is to the effect that among competing hypotheses that predict equally well, the hypothesis with the fewest assumptions should be chosen. Hence, the hypotheses of conspiracy theorists will not be chosen since they are often burdened with several assumptions. Nonetheless, it must be pointed out that Occam's razor is not an irrefutable principle of logic, and scholars are generally interested in two types of statements (hypotheses), namely statements of observations or existential statements that assert the existence of a singular entity; and universal statements that categorize all instances of a particular thing. The statements by bloggers or conspiracy theorists are often parsed in the latter form. They are universal statements and often include a false antecedent. It then becomes easy to raise questions about their veracity or to consider the statements vacuous given that the false antecedent prevents the use of the entire statements to infer anything about the truth of the other parts of the statements. Thus, it is unfortunate that the theorists seldom bother to demonstrate (albeit in a rigorous manner) how they inferred their universal statements from any number of singular existential statements.

It may be contended without any need for further inquiry that the answer to the question posed by Russ Winter about the healthy volunteers recruited for the clinical trial of TKM-Ebola would surely be in the report of the study. In the meantime, Russ Winter surmised that the volunteers were villagers in Guinea who were injected with the virus, unbeknownst to them, and then treated with the experimental drug. This is the false antecedent of his hypothesis. It is rather easy to assess the falsity of the claim given that it was made without any verification. Russ Winter justifies the claim with the assertion that WikiLeaks had revealed that homeless Polish people had been infected with Bird Flu in order to test the effectiveness of a vaccine. Thus, he used the perceived similarities between the Bird Flu virus and Ebola virus as the basis to infer some further similarity, viz., outbreaks of diseases caused by both viruses are due to the experimentation on unsuspecting people. One does not need John Stuart Mill's brain to submit that this is a false analogy given that the fact that both outbreaks are caused by viruses is not at all relevant to the question of whether Guinean villagers were injected with the Ebola virus in order to test TKM-Ebola.

In a three-part series on a blog in *Allvoices* (October 22, 2014), John-Thomas Didymus sought to establish (albeit without the favor of cogency) a link between a moratorium on funding from the federal government of the United States for research on the artificial modification (or weaponization) of disease pathogens (such as viruses) and the "biodefense-related research" conducted by The Consortium at the Kenema Government Hospital. The moratorium on federal funding applies to gain-of-function studies or projects that involve increasing the virulence of infections by viruses such as SARS, Flu, and MERS, as well as projects that seek to modify these viruses in order to ensure that they can infect humans. However, studies on naturally occurring viruses were not affected by the moratorium. These would include the studies on Lassa fever and other hemorrhagic fevers (such as Ebola) conducted in the Lassa Fever Ward of the Kenema Government Hospital.

Like Russ Winter, John-Thomas Didymus believes that since there is evidence of the modification of the Flu virus to one that may potentially infect humans, then surely the variant of the Zaire Ebola virus in West Africa is a "laboratory-engineered strain accidentally released from the US research laboratory." Despite the fact that attempts to increase the virulence of infections by the Flu virus show a clear disposition of researchers to weaponize viruses, this is also a false analogy. It would have been more logical to contend that given that the enactment of the moratorium was motivated by the artificial modification (or weaponization) of disease pathogens, it may be fair to assume that attempts have been made to weaponize the Ebola virus at some point; and American and European researchers are not forthcoming with information about when this may have happened. The furthest they have gone is accusing Russian researchers of attempting to weaponize the Ebola virus. Nonetheless, it is uncertain why existential import is assumed in this case. It is an existential fallacy to presuppose that all disease pathogens (including the Ebola virus) have been modified (weaponized) without evidence to this effect. John-Thomas Didymus believes the claim that the Ebola virus has been artificially modified has existential import because the researchers from Tulane University conducted biodefense-related studies at the Kenema Government Hospital between 2011 and 2014. He also claims that the USAMRIID that operates a Biosafety Level 4 facility in Fort Detrick conducted biodefense research on Ebola between 2006 and 2014. He then intimates that this broad-based partnership (The Consortium) prioritizes pathogens that are "classified as a potential bioterrorism threat."

On a blog of *The Daily Observer*, Monrovia (September 09, 2014), Cyril Broderick, Professor of Plant Pathology, was emphatic that the Ebola virus is a genetically modified organism. His statement is however based on Leonard Horowitz's controversial theory that the

AIDS and Ebola viruses originate from the deliberate infection of monkeys with the viral genes of other animals. Broderick further states that UN Agencies, including the WHO, have enticed some African countries to endorse the testing regimes, as well as the smokescreen created by promoting vaccinations. He then enjoins African countries to take legal actions against the institutions involved in the research and stop the use of wide-eyed and unwitting Africans as the subjects of testing.

However, Cyril Broderick's article is largely based on the essay by Jon Rappoport published on the *Global Research* site on August 02, 2014. Jon Rappoport raises a pertinent question about the presence of biological warfare researchers in Sierra Leone, Liberia, and Guinea, prior to the outbreak of the Ebola virus disease in these countries. The researchers belonged to the component institutions of The Consortium. He notes that researchers from Tulane University had stated that one of the objectives of their study in the region was to explore the future of viruses as bioweapons. He cites two releases by the University in 2007 and 2012 supporting this statement. He also cites a statement by the Sierra Leonean Ministry of Health and Sanitation published on its Facebook page on July 23, 2014, that laid out emergency measures that were to be taken. Amongst these measures is an exhortation to "Tulane University to stop Ebola testing during the current Ebola outbreak."

I was able to retrieve the statement published by the Ministry of Health and Sanitation on its Facebook page. It was to the effect that as of July 23, 2014, there had been 427 confirmed cases and 144 confirmed deaths. The Ministry also noted that the treatment centers in Kenema and Kailahun were attending to 65 patients suffering from the disease. This was less than 20 percent of the total number of confirmed cases at the time, implying that the burden of the Kenema Government Hospital had been significantly lessened by the middle of 2014. This may be due to the fact that the Ministry of Health and Sanitation and the WHO had since established the Ebola Emergency Operations Center (EOC), which served as the command and control center for the response activities. The statement published by the Ministry was motivated by the recommendations put forward by the EOC. The latter had asked for the relocation of the treatment center in Kenema to a more suitable location due to the loud requests by health workers and the town dwellers. The Ministry's statement ended with a note of ironic optimism to the effect that Sheikh Umar Khan was still alive and responding to treatment. This seemed to presage the death of the popular physician. Nonetheless, the most pertinent recommendation was that Tulane University should "stop Ebola testing during the current Ebola outbreak." That was the 4th recommendation put forward by the EOC. The recommendation logically begs a couple of questions that Jon Rappoport asks: why stop the testing? Were the results of the testing not helpful? Did the testing endanger the public?

Interestingly, the Ministry of Health and Sanitation said stop Ebola testing *during* the current outbreak. It is uncertain whether this implies that the Ministry had sanctioned research on Ebola by Tulane University prior to the outbreak, and it was advising the latter to cease the "Ebola testing" during the outbreak. Although Jon Rappoport does not attempt to provide unsubstantiated answers to these important questions, an almost irresistible yearning to most conspiracy theorists, he loudly wonders whether Tulane University researchers and their associates (The Consortium) had tested experimental treatments by injecting monoclonal antibodies into unwitting participants in the region affected by the outbreak. He also advises governments of the affected countries to investigate the vaccination campaigns prior to the Ebola outbreak by testing the vials of vaccines that were introduced into their citizens.

## THE CONSORTIUM: OFFICIAL PROFILE

A review of the information on The Consortium's website, as well as the websites of its component institutions and the publications of its researchers, should logically provide answers to the many questions raised by bloggers or conspiracy theorists. Nonetheless, as will be shown below this proves to be true only in part. On its website, The Consortium is said to be a partnership of research institutes that seek to promote health and safety around the world by creating new diagnostic procedures and therapies and reducing the incidence of viral hemorrhagic fevers. It is however noted that emphasis is placed on understanding the parts of the Lassa virus that may be recognized by the immune system. They evaluate antibodies from patients that have recovered from the disease and seek to determine whether the antibodies may help in developing a vaccine or therapeutics. Equally, the motivation for placing emphasis on Lassa fever is discussed. It has the highest incidence of any viral hemorrhagic fever and causes over 5,000 deaths each year across West Africa. The countries most affected are those of the Mano River Union, namely Sierra Leone, Liberia, and Guinea. The Consortium also notes that it intends to expand its research program to include other infectious agents such as Marburg and Ebola "that are of great concern to public health and bioterrorism."

The Consortium was established in 2010 following a five-year-contract between Tulane University and the National Institute of Allergy and Infectious Diseases (NIAID). The latter is part of the National Institutes of Health (NIH). Under the contract, the NIAID awarded US$15 million to Tulane University. As noted above, the government of the United States decided not to renew this funding in August 2014, during the Ebola crisis, without stating the motivation for the decision. Notwithstanding, The Consortium comprises seven other main partners, including Scripps Research Institute, Harvard

University/Broad Institute, University of California, Autoimmune Technologies LLC, Corgenix Medical Corporation, Irrua Specialist Teaching Hospital, Kenema Government Hospital, and University of Texas Medical Branch. Each partner plays a distinct role, and it may be important to examine these roles briefly.

## TULANE UNIVERSITY

Prior to the 2010 contract between NIAID and Tulane University, the latter had been involved in the treatment and prevention of Lassa fever. It may logically be assumed that the NIAID awarded US$15 million to the University because of its commendable effort in fighting this deadly disease that is endemic and threatens hundreds of thousands of lives in several countries on the West African coast. However, on the University's (School of Medicine – Lassa Fever Research) website, it is stated that Lassa fever is "classified as a potential bioterrorism threat." It is further stated that the causative agent of the fever is "classified as a Biosafety Level 4 (BSL-4) and NIAID Biodefense category A agent" due to its potential for aerosol release and ability to spread easily by human-human contact. It is noted further that the virus may be potentially used as a biological weapon directed against civilian or military targets, and it is important to develop counter-threat measures, including vaccines, therapeutics, and diagnostic assays. It is then noted that the University has established research programs in three West African countries, namely Sierra Leone, Guinea, and Nigeria, which provide clinical and laboratory resources for the studies on viral hemorrhagic fever. It was expected that the research programs would identify novel B cell epitopes on the virus proteins and help in understanding antibody-mediated protection in humans infected with the virus.

As such, Tulane University itself seems to assert that it effectively conducted biodefense-related studies at the Kenema Government

Hospital between 2010 and 2014. It also seems to insinuate that the NIAID's interest in the research project (and the motivation for awarding $15 million) is related to the fact that the Lassa virus is a Biosafety Level 4 (BSL-4) and NIAID Biodefense category A agent that may potentially be used as a biological weapon directed against civilian or military targets. In this light, it may be assumed that the NIAID sought to ensure that Tulane University developed counter-threat measures such as vaccines, therapeutics, and diagnostic assays. It is uncertain whether they have achieved this goal. Nonetheless, what is certain (at least officially) is that Tulane University was not involved in the artificial modification of the Ebola virus. There is no information to that effect on the School of Medicine's website, and I was unable to find any publication by any of the School's researchers that discusses the modification of the Ebola virus or the Lassa virus. On The Consortium's website, it is simply stated that Tulane University provided full equipped immunology and virology laboratories that were run by Drs Robinson, Garry, and Bausch.

## SCRIPPS RESEARCH INSTITUTE

It was founded in 1924 by Ellen Browning Scripps and set up to diagnose, treat, and investigate disorders of metabolism such as diabetes. It was initially part of Scripps Memorial Hospital that was founded in the same year. They separated in 1946. Over the years, it has recruited renowned researchers such as A. Baird Hastings (basic science), Frank Dixon (immunology), Frank Huennekens (biochemistry), Richard Lerner (molecular biology), Michael A. Marletta (biochemistry), and James Poulson (cell and molecular biology). Nine current and former faculty members, as well as members of its board of scientific governors, have been Nobel Prize laureates. One would be hard-pressed to find a more prestigious research institute. On its website, it states that it has led several seminal studies, and some examples are given. Although there is nothing on Lassa fever, it notes that researchers of the Institute (Andrew Ward and Erica Ollmann Saphire) have sought to identify weak spots on the surface of the Ebola virus that are targeted by the antibodies in the experimental drug cocktail, ZMapp. This was administered to many patients during the 2014 outbreak in West Africa. The objective of the study was to ascertain ways of developing an even better immunotherapeutic cocktail. It is further noted that this study is part of The Consortium's project to test antibodies from 25 laboratories around the world with the objective of formulating the best cocktail for neutralizing the Ebola virus. Hence, The Consortium seeks to study the new antibodies from human survivors of the 2014 outbreak. This implies that since the outbreak of the Ebola virus disease in West Africa, the main objective of The Consortium has been to evaluate antibodies from patients that have recovered from the disease and determine whether the antibodies may help in developing a vaccine or therapeutics. This suggests a shift from the emphasis on Lassa fever to the Ebola virus disease due to the 2014 outbreak. However, there is nothing to suggest that the researchers from Scripps that worked with The Consortium conducted any studies on the Ebola virus disease *prior to* the outbreak.

On The Consortium's website, Ollmann Saphire is presented as the researcher from Scripps that was most involved in The Consortium's research. She had a fully equipped laboratory wherein she looked into the production of antibodies that play important roles in the pathogenesis of hemorrhagic fever viruses. The findings of her work were said to provide information that is very crucial to the design of vaccines and inhibitors against the viruses. It is also stated that the findings would provide structural templates that would enable the other researchers of The Consortium to anticipate and respond swiftly to newly emerging and "man-made versions of the virus and viral proteins." It is uncertain what is meant by "man-made versions of the virus;" whether The Consortium implies that there is an existing threat posed by viruses that have been artificially modified or weaponized. It is also uncertain whether the findings of Ollmann Saphire's work were intended to provide information seminal only to the response to emerging versions of the Lassa virus. The Consortium talked of the production of antibodies that play important roles in the pathogenesis of hemorrhagic fever viruses, not just of the Lassa virus. Thus, one may not gainsay the Marburg and Ebola viruses were completely out of the frame. Nonetheless, even if Ollmann Saphire's research focused only on the Lassa virus, the statement that the findings of her research would provide structural templates that would enable other researchers to respond to newly emerging and "man-made versions of the virus" attests to the fact that there are effectively man-made versions of the Lassa virus out there. This is consistent with the contention that The Consortium was involved in biodefense-related research *prior* to the outbreak of the Ebola virus disease in West Africa. Notwithstanding, there is nothing to suggest that The Consortium sanctioned the artificial modification (or weaponization) of disease pathogens.

Michael Oldstone of Scripps equally collaborated with The Consortium. He is a pioneer in viral immunology and has published widely on viral pathogenesis and immunity. Oldstone focused on how viruses infect cells and seize control away from the immune system in order to establish persistent infections. He essentially looked at how three negative-strand viruses interacted with the immune, nervous and pulmonary system of the host: choriomeningitis, influenza, and measles.

From the above, it may be concluded that no researcher from Scripps conducted any studies on Ebola *prior to* the 2014 outbreak. As noted above, according to the Institute's website, it is after the outbreak that Andrew Ward and Erica Ollmann Saphire sought to identify weak spots on the surface of the Ebola virus that are targeted by the antibodies in the experimental drug cocktail, ZMapp. Seven patients who received the drug cocktail survived, and Ward and Saphire have since sought to demonstrate whether it may have been effective in these cases. They note that two ZMapp antibodies bind near the base of the virus and seem to prevent the virus from entering cells, while a third ZMapp antibody binds near the top of the virus and seems to alert the host's immune system as regards the site of infection. Ollmann Saphire is stated on the Institute's website as hoping that they may also develop another cocktail that would prevent mutant viruses from entering cells. This ties in with her role in The Consortium to provide structural templates that would enable her fellow researchers to anticipate and swiftly respond to newly emerging and man-made versions of the Lassa virus and viral proteins. Nonetheless, emphasis will be placed on the Ebola virus and not the Lassa virus. Also, from the information available to the public, it may be presumed that these researchers did not work with or develop a cocktail that would prevent "man-made versions" of the Ebola virus from entering cells since there is no statement to this effect. Given the nature of her study, it may, however, be submitted that The Consortium was officially involved in biodefense-related research (on Lassa fever) *prior* to the outbreak of the Ebola virus disease in West Africa.

## HARVARD UNIVERSITY / BROAD INSTITUTE

The Consortium's website notes that the Broad Institute and the FAS Center for Systems Biology provide the expertise on methods of evolutionary adaptation in pathogens and humans. The work is conducted at the Sabeti Laboratory that is named after Pardis Sabeti, Assistant Professor at the Department of Organismic and Evolutionary Biology and an Institute Member of Broad Institute and MIT. She is a computational geneticist and has conducted studies on analytical methods of detecting and investigating the evolution in the genomes of humans and other species, as well as the viral genetic factors that drive disease susceptibility to diseases such as Ebola and Lassa fever. She was actively involved in the fight against the Ebola virus disease following the 2014 outbreak and was one of the Ebola fighters named 'Person of the Year' by TIME Magazine. There is no evidence that she worked directly on Ebola *prior to* the outbreak. The only publication on the Sabeti Laboratory's website to this effect is a 2014 publication on the origin and transmission of the Ebola virus. This paper was published with a bevy of researchers, including Stephen Gire as lead researcher. The paper is discussed in Chapter 3. Two years earlier, Pardis Sabeti was part of a team (that comprised mostly Nigerian researchers) that published on molecular diagnostics for Lassa fever. The study was conducted at the Irrua Specialist Teaching Hospital, which also works with The Consortium. She was also part of a team that published a paper in 2012 on the selection of genes implicated in Lassa fever. This is further evidence that she was working on Lassa fever prior to the Ebola virus disease outbreak of 2014.

It is stated on The Consortium's website that the researchers at the Sabeti Laboratory are currently examining the genetic diversity of pathogens, and seek to ascertain how pathogens rapidly evolve. They also seek to identify the molecular basis of infectious diseases and define the components that enable pathogens to cause disease. It is expected that their research will help in the development of vaccines and more effective therapeutics. Given that there are researchers from a wide array of disciplines involved in the study, they should be able to combine several experimental and theoretical approaches in order to achieve their research objectives.

## CORGENIX MEDICAL CORPORATION

Founded in 1990, this institution has become a leader in the medical diagnostic industry. The ideal as stated on the institution's website is to conduct extensive research and provide comprehensive and effective products that will enhance health care around the globe. It currently sells more than 70 diagnostic products to hospitals, laboratories, and research institutes in different parts of the world. It is especially known for providing state-of-the-art in vitro diagnostic products for the detection and prevention of diseases. The company boasts of its strategic alliances and partnerships with esteemed researchers and research institutes around the world. One of such partnerships is of course with The Consortium. Corgenix was required to develop immunodiagnostic assays to detect Lassa fever. They were also supposed to make commercial grade ELISA that was configured with mutant Lassa fever virus proteins for quantifying B cell responses to diverse epitopes.

However, like other partners of The Consortium, Corgenix seems to have shifted focus from Lassa fever to the Ebola virus disease. In December 2014, it received $818,000 from the Bill & Melinda Gates Foundation and the Paul G. Allen Family Foundation to advance the development of a rapid diagnostic kit for Ebola. The subcontractors on the project include Tulane University, Autoimmune Technologies, and Zalgen Labs, all members of The Consortium. The President and CEO of Corgenix noted that the scope of the Ebola virus disease outbreak in West Africa led to an increased urgency to develop effective test kits. At present, test samples have to be sent to special laboratories several days away. The testing also requires special biohazard handling. Corgenix notes that its test kit would be used both in clinical and field laboratories and would enable healthcare professionals to diagnose patients in a matter of minutes. It would, therefore, eliminate the loss of time to diagnose and treat patients and thereby enhance the "response to public health and *bioterrorism threats* posed by the deadly virus."

It is strange that focus is placed on the 'bioterrorism threats' posed by the Ebola virus when there is no evidence of the existence of artificially modified forms of the virus or acknowledgment of the fact that some researchers are working on the modification. Nonetheless, the test kit would be developed along the same lines as the ReLASV rapid diagnostic test for the Lassa fever virus. This is further evidence of the fact that The Consortium was effectively working on enhancing the public health response to the Lassa virus before the 2014 outbreak of the Ebola virus disease. However, the focus is largely on Ebola at present.

## AUTOIMMUNE TECHNOLOGIES LLC

This is a producer of antigens and monoclonal and polyclonal antibodies that were used by other researchers of The Consortium. Many of its products are based on research findings and proprietary technologies that it has licensed from the School of Medicine of Tulane University. That was the purpose of its creation in 1995. Since then the company has explored disease mechanisms and examined therapies for autoimmune diseases. Together with Tulane University, it is currently seeking to develop anti-viral drugs (using its entry-inhibiting peptide technology) that are designed to prevent particles of a virus from fusing with their target cells. Peptides have been designed to inhibit the viruses that cause Influenza, HIV-1, measles, MERS/SARS, Dengue fever, and West Nile fever. The company's products target the following: Influenza, Lupus, Fibromyalgia Syndrome, Breast Cancer, and Gulf War Syndrome. It has not developed any drugs for Lassa fever, as well as for the Ebola virus disease. Nonetheless, together with other members of The Consortium, it received £2.9 million from the NIH as sub-awardees in order to enhance the Ebola Virus Diagnostic Tests. The prime grant award was made to Corgenix.

It is important to note that unlike Harvard University (Broad Institute and Sabeti Laboratory), Autoimmune Technologies *conducted studies on Ebola prior the 2014 outbreak.* In a press release, dated *April 14, 2010*, it announced that the NIH had awarded $600,000 to Corgenix for the extension of the collaborative effort to fight important viral diseases. The research institutes that collaborated with Corgenix under the grant included Autoimmune Technologies, Tulane University, and Scripps; all members of The Consortium. Autoimmune Technologies' Chief Science Officer, Russell B. Wilson, is noted in the press release as stating that the expected outcome of the study was the development of cost-effective and user-friendly tests for detecting the Ebola and Marburg viruses. He noted further that the resulting diagnostics would be crucial for the development of vaccines and other treatment modalities for the currently incurable diseases caused by these viruses. The President and CEO of Corgenix on his part intimated that they had the advantage of building on the very successful Lassa virus program and could in this light easily develop cutting edge diagnostic tests for Ebola and Marburg viruses on several delivery platforms. Lastly, Robert F Garry, Professor of Microbiology and Immunology at Tulane University, also expressed his satisfaction with the results of the collaborative effort between Corgenix, Autoimmune Technologies, Tulane University, and Scripps over the past five years. He noted that the diagnostic products for Lassa fever have been shown to be very effective in clinical settings in affected regions in Africa and would certainly have a meaningful impact on health care in that part of the globe. He then added that these diagnostic products would fill a gaping hole in *bioterrorism* defense. Interestingly, he used the term "critical gap" (not gaping hole), which may be confused with 'loophole.' Given that there is no reason to believe that he was referring to some ambiguity or uncertainty in the law on bioterrorism, the term "critical gap" here should be understood as implying a gaping hole in the extant literature. Notwithstanding, Robert F Garry intimated further that with the new NIH grant, they were going to expand the Lassa virus program to address two additional infectious agents which have the potential to kill scores of humans, and were naturally of concern to those in charge of maintaining a high level of *bioterrorism* preparedness. It may then be concluded that the above institutions adopted a two-pronged strategy: first, develop vaccines and other treatment modalities for the currently incurable diseases; and secondly, help in maintaining the level of bioterrorism preparedness.

As noted above, the two additional infectious agents that were examined are the Ebola and Marburg viruses. Autoimmune Technologies' press release dated April 14, 2010, therefore, proves without a shadow of a doubt that The Consortium was carrying out studies on Ebola prior to the outbreak of 2014. The press release even noted that the Ebola and Marburg viruses are characterized as Biosafety Level 4 agents because they present "a high individual risk of aerosol-transmitted laboratory infections" and are "agents which cause severe to fatal diseases for which vaccines or drugs are not available." As such, the extension of the collaborative effort within The Consortium to fight important viral diseases included enhancing the defense systems of their countries of origin against a bioterrorist attack involving the use of the Ebola virus. It is uncertain whether the researchers conducted studies on the Zaire Ebola virus or the Cote d'Ivoire Ebola virus or the Sudan Ebola virus. The outbreak in 2014 in parts of West Africa was caused by the Zaire Ebola virus. It is also uncertain whether this is what the Ministry of Health and Sanitation of Sierra Leone referred to as "Ebola testing" in the statement it published on July 23, 2014. If that was the case then why did the Ministry of Health and Sanitation use the word "testing" which may be interpreted as meaning the use of measures to reveal the strengths or capabilities of the vaccines or treatments developed? Also, if that was the case, it may be important to ask why the "testing" was conducted in West Africa where there is a no Biosafety Level 4 laboratory wherein researchers could play with agents that present "a high individual risk of aerosol-transmitted laboratory infections."

## UNIVERSITY OF TEXAS MEDICAL BRANCH

This branch was established in 1891 as the Medical Department of the University of Texas. At the time it had only 23 students and 13 faculty members. It was Texas' first academic health center and opened the first schools of medicine and nursing in the state. Today it boasts of more than 2500 students and over 1000 faculty members. It comprises several hospitals and clinics that provide primary and specialized health care, as well as research facilities. Of concern here is the Department of Microbiology and Immunology that is at the forefront of the development of new knowledge on the complex relationship between human health and disease and microbiological and immunological processes. On the Department's website, it is stated that it seeks cures for common and emerging infectious diseases. The pathogens listed include salmonella, anthrax, HIV, and West Nile virus. It also boasts about its Biosafety Levels 3 and 4 containment laboratories. This implies that they have laboratories in which work is done with pathogens that may cause serious or potentially fatal disease through aerosol-transmitted infections. Level 4 is required for work with dangerous pathogens such as Marburg virus, Lassa virus, and Ebola virus.

The Consortium's man at the University of Texas Medical Branch works in the Galveston National Laboratory, a Biosafety Level 4 containment laboratory. This is the only operational Biosafety Level 4 containment laboratory on a university campus in the United States. He is Thomas Geisbert and was also a TIME Magazine's 2014 Person of the Year. He is one of the five Ebola experts at the University. In fact, the University's website notes that Thomas Geisbert has studied the Ebola virus for more than two decades and spent several years working with the United States Army Medical Research Institute of Infectious Disease at Fort Detrick. In March of 2014, he was awarded (together with Profectus Biosciences, Tekmira Pharmaceuticals, and

Vanderbilt University Medical Center) $26 million (to be distributed over five years) by the NIH to "advance treatments of the highly lethal hemorrhagic fever viruses Ebola and Marburg." The University's website at the time noted that these filoviruses are classified "Tier 1" pathogens by the Department of Health and Human Services because "they are considered agents with the highest risk of being *deliberately misused by bioterrorists* to cause mass casualties and produce devastating effects to the economy, critical infrastructure, and public confidence." Thomas Geisbert and the other recipients were therefore expected to develop and test new vaccines and treatments. James E. Crowe Jr of Vanderbilt University Medical Center noted that they would seek to delineate the mechanisms by which naturally occurring antibodies kill Ebola and Marburg viruses in order to ascertain a rational vaccine design and testing. He noted further that they were using human monoclonal antibodies that were derived from the blood cells of naturally infected human survivors to develop vaccines and cures. He did not state whether the infected human survivors were volunteers or patients at a medical center. Nonetheless, it would be presumptuous to suggest that he was talking about unwitting volunteers in such an open forum.

The researchers were expected to conduct three interdependent studies supported by the Biosafety Level 4 Galveston National Laboratory. In August of 2014, Thomas Geisbert intimated that a blend of three monoclonal antibodies (ZMAPP) could completely protect monkeys against a lethal dose of Ebola within five days of exposure. Clinical signs of the disease can be seen already by this time. This was a marked improvement from a previous blend of small interfering RNAs and antibodies that had to be administered within two days of infection. The blend of three monoclonal antibodies was so successful that all the animals survived, and none showed any evidence of the virus in their systems after 21 days. ZMAPP, therefore, inhibited the replication of the virus in the cell culture. Thomas Geisbert noted that several patients had been given ZMAPP following the Ebola outbreak in West Africa, and many survived, including two American healthcare workers. Nonetheless, he observed that it is uncertain whether ZMAPP effectively cured those patients given that 45% of patients during the outbreak survived without treatment, and two patients who were given ZMAPP (albeit well after the recommended deadline) did not survive. With regard to vaccines, he noted that the vesicular stomatitis virus (VSV)-based vaccines had completely protected monkeys against Ebola and Marburg infection. In 2015, he published several articles on the protection of primates by vaccines in *The Journal of Clinical Investigations*.

It goes without saying that this eminent researcher was conducting studies on the Ebola virus disease prior to the 2014 outbreak. Nonetheless, what is most intriguing is why an Ebola virus disease expert was involved with The Consortium when the latter has repeatedly claimed that its research prior to the outbreak was exclusively focused on the Lassa virus. The Consortium's website describes the status of the Ebola expert as "partner" although there was no reported case of Ebola in West Africa at the time The Consortium was set up. It states that Thomas Geisbert's research placed emphasis on the viruses that cause hemorrhagic fevers such as Lassa, Ebola, and Marburg. That is logical but does not explain the role of the Ebola expert. However, at the time of setting up The Consortium, there were no vaccines approved for use in humans against any of the three viruses. Thus, Thomas Geisbert's input was important given that he had shown that VSV-based vaccines could completely protect primates against viruses that cause Ebola and Marburg fevers. As such, it was important to modify the vaccine vector for optimal safety and immunogenicity, and also identify the antigens that should comprise a multiagent vaccine that could protect against different groups of hemorrhagic fever viruses. Notwithstanding, unlike The Consortium, the University of Texas Medical Branch's newsroom report gave the impression that Thomas Geisbert's research was exclusively focused on the Ebola and Marburg viruses. No mention was made of the Lassa virus.

## INSTITUTE OF MICROBIOLOGY OF
## UNIVERSITÉ DE LAUSANNE, SWITZERLAND

The diagnostic laboratory of this institute is very active in research and development, as well as applied research. The research conducted is largely focused on the diagnosis of infectious diseases. It generally provides microbiological diagnostics for hospitalized patients. The Consortium's contact within this institute is Stefan Kunz, Associate Professor of Microbiology. On the Institute's website, it is noted that its researchers have focused on arenaviruses which have emerged as causative agents of fatal diseases such as viral hemorrhagic fevers that are prevalent in Africa and South America. Thus, Stefan Kunz's role in The Consortium was to ascertain the ways in which viruses invade and shut down the anti-viral defense mechanisms of human cells. He placed particular emphasis on the Lassa virus. His team is still examining the interaction between arenaviruses and human cells in order to determine new ways of therapeutic intervention.

## ZALGEN LABS, LLC

This institution became operational in 2013. It was established by the Maryland Economic Development Corporation (MEDCO). One of the founders of the institution is Tulane University's Robert F. Garry, also a leading researcher of The Consortium. Zalgen Labs LLC focuses on the generation of recombinant proteins from "difficult-to-express" genes. The end goal is to contribute to the effective management of the Lassa fever. In this light, it has developed methods for the production of Lassa virus-like particles (VLP) that are essentially empty and non-infectious virions which contain all the important viral proteins in a quasi-native conformation. The institution believes the VLP may be the next generation vaccine platforms for the Lassa hemorrhagic fever. Its website talks of the demonstration of the efficacy of the first three human monoclonal antibodies in Biosafety Level-4 settings. It may be safe to assume it is referring to Thomas Geisbert's team's use of human monoclonal antibodies that were derived from the blood cells of naturally infected human survivors to develop vaccines and cures. Nonetheless, the latter talked about vaccines and cures for Ebola and Marburg fevers, while Zalgen Labs LLC seems to focus on Lassa fever. Likewise James E. Crowe Jr of Vanderbilt University Medical Center, Zalgen Labs LLC does not state whether the human monoclonal antibodies were hatched from volunteers.

## IRRUA SPECIALIST TEACHING HOSPITAL (ISTH)

Like the Kenema Government Hospital, the ISTH does not contribute (at least intellectually) to the research on the effective ways of managing the hemorrhagic fevers. There are no researchers from the ISTH working on the delineation of the mechanisms by which naturally occurring antibodies kill Ebola, Lassa, and Marburg viruses in order to ascertain vaccine designs and testing. The importance of the ISTH is purely logistical. It is located in the State of Edo in Nigeria, a hotspot of Lassa fever. It receives patients from the neighboring Delta, Kogi, and Ondo States that are affected by Lassa fever. The ISTH hosts the Institute of Lassa Fever Research and Control (ILFRC). The latter institute was established in 2007 and took over the activities of the Lassa Fever Control Committee, which was set up by the Nigerian Ministry of Health in 2001. The Committee worked closely with the University of Maiduguri Teaching Hospital and the Federal Medical Centre of Owerri. The main objectives were to establish a center of excellence in rural and sub-urban medicine, and effectively manage viral hemorrhagic fevers. Nonetheless, despite the ambition as regards viral hemorrhagic fevers, no researcher from the Institute has contributed directly to the studies undertaken by The Consortium.

It is interesting that no mention is made of The Consortium on the ILFRC's poorly designed website. Equally, it does not talk of the study site established by The Consortium. There are a couple of pictures of Robert F. Gary of Tulane University on the website (partnerships page) which suggests that the institution's association with The Consortium may be limited to Robert F. Gary's relationship with the management of the ISTH. Thus, the ILFRC's website talks about the partnership between the management of the ISTH and the Bernhard Nocht Institute for Biology, as well as Harvard University, Tulane University, Lahor Research Laboratory, and the Public Health Center. It also talks about the partnership between ISTH and Rare and Imported Pathogens Department, HPA Microbiology Services, and Porton Down. The latter partnership seeks to investigate pathogens that cause diseases that show clinical resemblance to Lass fever but are PCR negative for the Lassa virus.

## CONCERNS RAISED BY 'CONSPIRACY' THEORISTS

Some of the concerns of the 'conspiracy theorists' or bloggers were discussed above. It was noted that some of these concerns are pertinent while others are inapposite. Nonetheless, there is no denying that the concerns are largely expressed within the frame of a grand theory of researchers colluding to conduct experimental treatments on wide-eyed and unwitting participants in the region affected by the outbreak of the Ebola virus disease. Despite the absence of evidence of collusion, it would be foolhardy to dismiss the concerns of these theorists outright given the pertinence of a few. Thus, the fact that the conspiracy theorists made a hasty conclusion about a collusion without considering all variables does not in itself invalidate all of their questions or discredit all of their claims.

It is shown above that in addition to the evidence of the modification of the Flu virus to one that may potentially infect humans, researchers of The Consortium have intimated that there are "man-made versions" of viruses and viral proteins out there. Nonetheless, this is not evidence of the existence of a "laboratory-engineered strain" of the Ebola virus that may have been "accidentally released from the US research laboratory in Sierra Leone." It is only fair to assume that the Ebola virus may have been modified at some point, and American and European researchers are not forthcoming with information about when this may have happened. Nonetheless, they have accused Russian researchers of attempting to weaponize the Ebola virus.

It is also shown above that the researchers from Tulane University effectively conducted biodefense-related studies at the Kenema Government Hospital between 2011 and 2014. Also, it is noted that the USAMRIID effectively operates a Biosafety Level 4 facility in Fort Detrick in which biodefense research has been conducted. Also, it is shown that The Consortium prioritized pathogens that are classified as potential bioterrorism threats, including the Marburg and Ebola viruses. Thus, some researchers of The Consortium effectively carried out studies on the Ebola virus disease prior to the 2014 outbreak of the disease in parts of West Africa. Equally, there were Ebola experts working with The Consortium prior to the outbreak, despite the fact that emphasis was allegedly placed on Lassa fever. These facts raised by the conspiracy theorists are true and beg many questions, although they do not in any way constitute evidence and cannot support the claim that the Ebola virus had been artificially modified by researchers of The Consortium prior to the 2014 outbreak. Equally, they do not support the claim that the outbreak was caused by a human clinical trial that got out of control. The human clinical trial carried out by Tekmira is relatively well documented, although many questions related to the Phase I trial remain unanswered.

## HUMAN CLINICAL TRIAL BY TEKMIRA

It was expected that Phase I of the trial would guide the researchers working with and for Tekmira in determining the appropriate dose of TKM-Ebola for potential use as a medical countermeasure against the Ebola virus, and possibly other hemorrhagic fever viruses. In a press release, Mark J. Murray, the President and CEO of Tekmira had noted that the results of the trial would be published in the second half of 2014. However, the company did not publish the findings as promised because, in July 2014, the FDA put the trial on clinical hold on the Investigational New Drug application (IND) in order to obtain additional information and effectively assess the effect of the drug. The FDA had initially granted Tekmira a Fast Track designation for the development of the drug. During the clinical hold, the multiple ascending dose phase of the trial was modified in order to ensure the safety of healthy volunteers. The hold was then modified to a partial hold in order to administer the drug to patients with confirmed or suspected infection. In April 2015, the FDA again modified the hold in order to permit Tekmira to repeat dosing of healthy individuals. The threshold was 0.24mg/kg/day in healthy individuals. The company surprisingly resumed the clinical trial with Phase II without publishing the findings of Phase I. It then announced that the findings of Phase II would be published in the second half of 2015.

However, on June 19, 2015, Tekmira released a press statement to the effect that the Phase II of the human clinical trial of TKM-Ebola-Guinea had reached a predefined statistical endpoint and enrollment had been closed. As pointed out by Andrew Pollack of *The New York Times* (June 19, 2005), the experimental drug had not worked on patients in Sierra Leone. Tekmira noted in the statement that the drug "was not likely to demonstrate an overall therapeutic benefit" even if enrollment continued. Interestingly, the company did not publish its findings and simply said that data was still being analyzed. It equally did not publish the long-awaited findings of Phase I of the clinical trial although it had promised to do so in the second half of 2015. Peter Horby of Oxford University, the chief investigator on the study (Phase II), told *The New York Times* that more time was needed to analyze the data. *The New York Times* said the trial was conducted in Sierra Leone and sponsored by a biomedical research charity based in the UK, the Wellcome Trust. For ethical reasons, the researchers did not use a control group of patients receiving a placebo or a different drug. All the patients were given the experimental drug. The Phase II single arm trial was referred to as the Rapid Assessment of Potential Interventions and Drugs for Ebola (RAPIDE).

It is interesting that Tekmira's press release talked of TKM-Ebola-Guinea and not simply TKM-Ebola. TKM-Ebola-Guinea is an anti-Ebola RNAi therapeutic that targets the Ebola-Guinea strain or more specifically, the Zaire Ebola virus (Makona variant), which diverges slightly from the Kikwit strain that was the original target of the drug. The Makona strain was responsible for the outbreak in parts of West Africa in 2014, while the Kikwit strain was responsible for the outbreak in the Democratic Republic of Congo (previously known as Zaire). As mentioned above, the press release in 2014 talked of TKM-Ebola. Thus, it may be assumed that the Phase I of the human clinical trial was conducted in an undisclosed location using TKM-Ebola, while the Phase II of the trial (sponsored by Wellcome Trust) was conducted in Sierra Leone in the middle of the epidemic using the TKM-Ebola-Guinea. As such, there is still so much uncertainty about the Phase I of the trial: where was it conducted, and where were the healthy volunteers recruited. It is also uncertain whether the order by the Sierra Leonean Ministry of Health and Sanitation to Tulane University (The Consortium) to "stop Ebola testing" was one of the reasons that motivated the decision to discontinue the trial; apart from the fact that Phase III (administering the drug to large groups of people) was "not likely to demonstrate an overall therapeutic benefit." The publication of the findings of Phases I and II of the trial would certainly help clarify these concerns, and it is only unfortunate that so much time is required to analyze the data.

On October 1, 2015, I reached out via email to Peter Horby of Oxford University, the chief investigator on the Phase II study. My mail read as follows:

*Dear Prof Horby,*

*I am currently carrying out a study on the media reports of 2014 outbreak of the Ebola virus disease in parts of West Africa, as well as the information that trickled down to West African citizens and their reactions.*

*In this light, I would be very grateful if you can shed some light on the clinical trials conducted by Tekmira using TKM-Ebola and TKM-Ebola-Guinea. This is because the findings of these trials are yet to be published. On January 14, 2014, it was announced that Tekmira had dosed first subjects in a Phase I human clinical trial of TKM-Ebola. However, the findings of this trial (where it was conducted, where the volunteers were recruited from, safe dosage, side effects, etc.) were never published. The trial had resumed after the clinical hold put by the FDA.*

*Also, on June 19, 2015, Tekmira released a press statement to the effect that the Phase II of the human clinical trial of TKM-Ebola-Guinea (not TKM-Ebola) had reached a predefined statistical endpoint and enrolment had been closed. Also, the findings of the Phase II trial have not been published. Is there a tentative date on when they might be published?*

*It is also uncertain whether Phase I of the trial using TKM-Ebola-Guinea was ever conducted; or whether Phase II using*

> *TKM-Ebola-Guinea was conducted on the basis of the results of the Phase I trial using TKM-Ebola.*
>
> *Lastly, did the Ministry of Health and Sanitation of Sierra Leone influence the decision to discontinue the trial in Sierra Leone?*
>
> *I would like to thank you again in advance for taking time out and clarifying the above.*
>
> *Kindest regards,*
> *Constantine N. Nana*

Peter Horby replied on October 02, 2015. He noted that the Phase II trial was discontinued because they had met a pre-defined statistical endpoint, and not due to any request from a Government or agency to stop. He also said the results of the trial had been submitted for publication. However, most intriguing, he said he had no information as regards the results of the Phase I trial.

It is clear from Peter Horby's correspondence that the order by the Sierra Leonean Ministry of Health and Sanitation to Tulane University (The Consortium) to "stop Ebola testing" was not one of the reasons that motivated the decision to discontinue the human clinical trial. It was stopped because they had met a pre-defined statistical endpoint or due to the fact that further research was unlikely to demonstrate an overall therapeutic benefit. Nonetheless, what is strange from Peter Horby's email is that the chief investigator on the Phase II study has no information about the Phase I study. Although the Phase II study simply implies that the experimental drug was given to a larger group of humans to determine its effectiveness and safety, one would have thought investigators on the Phase II study used the results of the Phase I study as premise; given that the findings of the Phase I study ought to have justified the carrying out of Phase II. If the drugs were neither effective nor safe following administration to a small group of humans during the Phase I study, it would have been unethical to proceed with Phase II. Thus, it is important to determine the results of the Phase I study and also confirm where the trial was conducted and who were the healthy volunteers used.

Notwithstanding, the findings of the preclinical study were published by Geisbert et al. in *The Lancet* (Volume 375, of May 29, 2010). They are to the effect that when siRNA targeting the Ebola virus was delivered using Tekmira's LNP technology, it provided 100 percent protection to previously infected non-human primates.

Also, Tekmira's press release in early 2014 briefly discussed the methodology employed and the nature of the therapeutic. It also briefly discussed the Biodefense Therapeutic Program of the United States Army, the RNA Interference Therapeutic (RNAi), and Tekmira LNP. It noted that the preclinical trial was randomized placebo-controlled and single-blind, and involved both single and multiple ascending doses of TKM-Ebola. There were four planned groups, each group comprising four subjects in the single dose arm of the trial; and three planned groups, each comprising four subjects in the multiple dose arm. Within each group, one subject received a placebo while the other three subjects received TKM-Ebola. It was expected that the trial would help the researchers evaluate the safety, tolerability, and pharmacokinetics of administering TKM-Ebola to healthy adults. Nonetheless, the article by Geisbert et al. does not specify where the preclinical study was conducted. Also, it is uncertain whether the Phase I of the ensuing human clinical trial using TKM-Ebola was conducted in Sierra Leone prior to the outbreak of the Ebola virus disease. Such disclosure would no doubt become a political hot potato.

The press release by Tekmira noted that TKM-Ebola was developed under a contract with the Department of Defense's Joint Project

Management Medical Countermeasure Systems (JPM-MCS). No mention is made of The Consortium or Tulane University. However, it noted that as part of the Joint Program Executive Office for Chemical and Biological Defense, JPM-MCS seeks to provide the military forces of the United States with "safe, effective and innovative medical solutions to counter chemical, biological, radiological and nuclear threats." It also noted that the project would enhance the biodefense response capability of the United States. As such, Tekmira was not testing a bioweapons agent but seeking a solution to counter the threat of such an agent. It may nonetheless be fair to contend that the Phase I human clinical trial using TKM-Ebola was part of the biodefense research.

Lastly, it is only fair to point out that the RNAi may also treat several other diseases that affect humans by inhibiting the expression of the genes that cause the diseases. It has been referred to in the past as co-suppression, quelling, and post-transcriptional gene silencing. A study published in 1998 on RNAi in the nematode worm Caenorhabditis elegans gave Andrew Fire and Craig Mello the 2006 Nobel Prize in Medicine. Given that the RNAi requires an effective technology for delivery, Tekmira has attempted to employ its LNP technology or the Stable Nucleic Acid-lipid Parties (SNALP). It contains many lipid components that may be adjusted in accordance with the application. It also provides uniform lipid nanoparticles with high efficiency that deliver the RNAi therapeutics to disease sites.

As such, Tekmira has certainly helped not only in enhancing the biodefense response capability of the United States, but also it attempts to treat diseases affecting humans generally. However, this does not imply that all its study techniques have been foolproof. The fact that very little is known about the Phase I of the human clinical trial using TKM-Ebola lends support to the bloggers' presentiment of collusion. Did the trial lead to a situation that got totally out of control, such as the outbreak of the Ebola virus disease?

# CHAPTER 3

# The Spillover Event

This event occurs when a virus spills over from one animal (reservoir) to another animal or human (a novel host). Thus, it occurs when an epidemic is caused in a new host population by a reservoir population. Sometimes referred to as the pathogen spillover, it is one of the most abstruse parts of the science of the causes and effects of diseases. Spillover events are as rare as they are important given that they are often followed by a new disease and therefore have the potential to cause major outbreaks. Also, many spillover events go unnoticed as many animal and human hosts often literally provide a dead end for the transmission of many diseases. Where the natural reservoir is unknown, the spillover event often becomes the upshot of speculation. A good example is the conjecture about bats infecting cave persons with mumps and measles. Richard Preston in his nonfiction thriller, *The Hot Zone*, talks about USAMRIID biohazard experts spending "years traveling across central Africa in search of the reservoirs of Ebola and Marburg viruses" but never finding the viruses in their natural hiding place. Thus, he concluded that no one knew where the viruses came from, and no one knew where they lived in nature since the trail always petered out in the forests or savannas of Africa.

David Quammen in his book *Ebola: The Natural and Human History of A Deadly Virus*, notes that the identity of the reservoir host of the Ebola virus remains one of the darkest little mysteries in the realm of infectious disease. He believes the mystery, along with various efforts to solve it, dates back to the first recognized emergence of the Ebola virus and the disease it caused in 1976. Saying the mystery dates back to the first recognized emergence of the virus and the disease may imply many things, including that the mystery may only be solved with information about the first incident and diagnoses. Since the only established pattern thus far is the sudden appearance of the virus and disease followed by sudden disappearance into thin air, it may be contended that the mystery is related to the first incidents and diagnoses of each outbreak. However, the lack of any information about the actual patient zero of an outbreak further mystifies the plot.

The above notwithstanding, the Ebola virus disease is no doubt one of the most perplexing of mysteries. There have been several recorded outbreaks since 1976 and yet in each case the lineage of the virus that caused the outbreak has disappeared, leaving no trace. David Quammen, therefore, describes the virus as "an evolutionary loser" that has been unable to find a way to become an endemic disease in human populations. Hence, he argues that every spillover event is a gamble by the virus to transcend the dead end. Nonetheless, it is uncertain why the virus would constantly seek to transfer to new hosts when it seems to have an unidentifiable cozy nook wherein it has lived and multiplied for heaven knows how long without being perturbed. However, the host-seeking behavior of these ancient life forms is well-established, and it is not always per logic. What is not well-established is why some viruses like the Ebola virus seem to appear out of nowhere and disappear into thin air after an uproar. There is no evidence that humans have disturbed their natural reservoirs by hunting them for meat or dragging them out of their ecosystems. This shows that unless it is the researcher that causes the virus to venture out into a new host, the researcher's postulate about the spillover event and outbreak would largely be based on speculation.

When researchers speculate, the result is often an opinion reached after careful consideration of facts, whereby the process can be verified. However, there is always the risk that the media would restate a conjectural contention based on inconclusive evidence as a fact. This is especially the case with conjectural contentions about the cause of a major outbreak. The statements about the cause of the disease are seldom as unequivocal in publications by researchers as it is in newspaper articles.

In 1982, a team of researchers at the Center for Disease Control and Prevention (CDC) led by William Darrow and David Auerbach published the findings of an epidemiologic study on the transmission pattern of HIV in the United States. The findings of an extended epidemiologic investigation across the United States were also published in an article in *The American Journal of Medicine* (No 76) two years later. The studies showed how an infected person referred to as 'Patient O' transmitted the virus to several partners, who in turn transmitted the virus to others. In 1987, Penguin published a book by Randy Shilts that was supposedly based on those findings. In the book, Randy named Gaetan Dugas, a Canadian flight attendant as 'Patient O.' However, in 1991, William Darrow claimed that the methods used in the epidemiologic study were flawed and that Randy Shilts had impudently misrepresented their findings. This implied that the story that Gaetan Dugas was the index case was nothing more than a myth born out of cynicism and media sensationalism. In 2007, Michael Worobey and Arthur Pitchenik developed a theory in a paper published in the *Proceedings of the National Academy of Sciences* that postulated the movement of HIV from Africa to Haiti and then to the United States around 1969 via a single immigrant. However, Robert Rayford, an American teenager who had never traveled outside the Midwestern United States died of complications from AIDS in 1969 and is suspected to have been infected around 1966. Thus, there were effectively carriers of HIV in the United States before the arrival of the hypothetical single immigrant from Haiti in Worobey's and Pitchenik's postulate.

From the above, it is clear that it is presumptuous to identify an individual as the index case in a disease outbreak without clear and convincing evidence. This is especially the case with diseases that are transmitted to humans through an animal reservoir and where it is likely that several other humans may have come into contact with the animal reservoir at an earlier date. An article by Denise Grady and Sheri Fink published on August 09, 2014 in *The New York Times*; and an article by Madison Park published on October 10, 2014, on CNN's website (amongst many others) stated that the outbreak of the Ebola virus disease in parts of West Africa might have started with a two-year-old child in a village in Guinea. Madison Park supports her statement with a citation of the article by Baize et al. published in *The New England Journal of Medicine* on August 09, 2014. As noted in Chapter 1, Baize et al. had concluded that "the suspected first case of the outbreak was a two-year-old child who died in Meliandou in Gueckedou prefecture on December 06, 2013." They provided a rather clear but hypothetical map of the transmission chains of the disease showing how it spread to the child's mother, sister, and grandmother, who all died; and then to the nurse and village midwife, and outside the village to the family member that took care of the village midwife, and several people who attended the grandmother's funeral.

However, Sylvain Baize was later on cited by Denise Grady and Sheri Fink (*The New York Times*) to the effect that there might have been an earlier case that went undiscovered, and it was almost impossible to explain how the two-year-old child could have become the first person infected. This implies that the reporters of *The New York Times* and CNN had simply interpreted the findings of Baize et al.'s work in the same way Randy Shilts had interpreted the findings of William Darrow's team's work some twenty-six years earlier. In both instances, the reporters presumptuously identified the index case on the basis of suppositions. This was done in total disregard of the consequences of their publication on the good reputation of the deceased and his family. In the case of the two-year-old child in Guinea, it was done irrespective of the child's family's indigence and unwitting assiduity. After all, how many people from the African wilderness have ever initiated proceedings for defamation against a European or American paper or publisher?

Suzanne Beukes of the South African *Daily Maverick*, which is part of the Guardian Network, wrote an article about her trip to the supposed Patient Zero's village, Meliandou. It was published on UNICEF's website on October 27, 2014, and on *The Guardian*'s website on October 28, 2014. To Suzanne Beukes' credit, she describes this village as "the heart of where Ebola is thought to have originated in West Africa." Hence, she chooses words to convey a message that although the outbreak is claimed to have started in Meliandou, there is no proof to this effect. However, this is the closest she came to telling her readers that the conjecture about the index case in Meliandou was merely a supposition made as a basis for further investigation, without any firm conviction that it represents the truth. She consistently calls Meliandou, "Ground Zero", and the two-year-old child, "Patient Zero." As an aside, she claims that every South African leaving the country for mainland Africa is quite apprehensive and fills their bag with disinfectants, non-contact thermometers, malaria tablets, gloves, face masks, and hand sanitizers. It is ironical that this is equally the state of mind of most Europeans and Americans visiting South Africa. Notwithstanding, her article vividly describes the village and provides a succinct account of the child's life. The discussion in the next section is based in part on her account.

## THE MEDIA'S INDEX CASE: EMILE OUAMONOU

In Meliandou, the adventurous Suzanne Beukes met a grieving inhabitant who sifted through a heap of pictures and drew out that of his deceased two-year-old child. Beukes describes the child as "the world's most unnamed toddler." She talks about the "precious face's" hobby and ghastly experience shortly before dying. The child, Emile Ouamonou, has unfortunately become the protagonist of the Ebola tragedy because for some unspecified reason some oblivious researchers and many impulsive journalists have decided to identify him as the index case or the first patient in the Ebola virus disease outbreak in parts of West Africa. It is uncertain why it has been so difficult to refer to the child simply as the point where the chains of transmission seemed to have ended as per the first epidemiologic study conducted shortly after the outbreak. In a matter of a few months, the child described by Baize et al. in the landmark article published in *The New England Journal of Medicine* as "the suspected first case of the outbreak" had simply become the established Patient Zero without any further evidence. Thus, for reasons unknown, journalists decided to start reporting a suspected case as the first laboratory-confirmed case. Interestingly, the article by Baize et al. is often cited as explaining how the researchers finally identified Patient Zero. Never mind that next to the diagram published by Baize et al. showing the putative transmission chains, it is noted that "Dashed arrows indicate that the epidemiologic links are not well-established" – and in the diagram only dashed arrows link the suspected cases and the laboratory-confirmed cases. Never mind that Baize et al. note as regards the clinical and epidemiologic analysis that a subsequent investigation confirmed the origin of the outbreak in Meliandou but revealed a different timing of early incidents "including the death of Patient S1 [Emile Ouamonou] at the end of December [2013], and the deaths of Patients S2 [Emile's sister], S3 [Emile's mother], and S4 [Emile's grandmother] in January [2014]." The initial investigation had revealed that Emile died on December 06, 2013.

Patient S7), died at the end of December 2013. This is also the case with a deceased patient identified as S8, who is said to have attended S4's funeral but died on January 30, 2014. If Patient Zero died in the last week of December 2013, then patients on the first link of the transmission chain should have died toward the end of January or in the first week of February, not in the first week of January 2014 (S4).

What is most interesting is that there was no confirmed case in Emile's village at the time the study was conducted. None of the infected individuals had for some reason infected some friend, lover or business partner. As regards previous outbreaks, the lineage of the virus that caused the outbreaks disappeared without a trace only after medical personnel had intervened and imposed isolation on ground zero for several months. In this case, the virus seemed to have disappeared only after about three or four months and without the intervention of any medical personnel. Also, Etienne Ouamonou, Emile's father was not infected although he had nursed his infected children shortly before they died. That is quite some exposure. It is noted in Chapter 1 that subsequent studies have revealed that some people may have an immune response to the Ebola virus given that they have never presented with symptoms after sustained exposure to the virus. However, if Etienne Ouamonou were one of them, the researchers would certainly have found it noteworthy, and that would have been cogent evidence that his family was killed by the Ebola virus.

Given the unreliability of the testimonies on the symptoms and ailments suffered by the patients (including the information on their death certificates), it may be difficult to determine whether some of the above patients did not suffer from Lassa fever which is endemic in the region and has similar symptoms to the Ebola virus disease. Apart from the father's testimony, there is nothing to suggest that vomiting, diarrhea, and fever were the prominent features of the ailment suffered by Emile and other deceased members of his family. It is also interesting that the healthcare professional saw black or bloody diarrhea and thought of cholera, although cholera-related diarrhea is often pale and milky. Hence, one may contend that the fact that the early researchers were investigating the origin of the Ebola virus disease may have subtly prompted them to focus on these symptoms, or they may have asked questions that contained information that they were looking to have confirmed. In a story published on *Zeit Online*, Etienne Ouamonou notes that several "foreigners" including physicians, biologists, and epidemiologists visited him shortly after the outbreak and asked many questions for days on end. The article also notes that it is from these visitors that Etienne first heard of the word "Ebola."

Nonetheless, despite the fact that there is still a strong case for arguing that Emile and the members of his family all died from the Ebola virus disease, it remains that the contention that Emile is Patient Zero awaits demonstration. First, it is uncertain whether he was not infected by his mother or grandmother. The fact that he allegedly died before the latter does not necessarily imply that he transmitted the virus to them. A study conducted by the WHO's Ebola Response Team found that the Ebola virus disease is most deadly among babies and toddlers. They get sick faster as the average incubation period is about seven days in babies but can be as long as 21 days in adults. As such, it is more likely that the two-year-old Emile picked up the virus from his 25-year-old mother or 46-year-old grandmother but died first since the incubation period is much shorter for babies and toddlers. His four-year-old sister died shortly after him.

The second reason why Emile is most certainly not Patient Zero is that he is least likely to have come into contact with the host or reservoir of the virus. The study by Baize et al. concluded that there was only a single introduction of the virus into the population in Meliandou due to the high degree of similarity among the gene sequences and the epidemiologic links between the cases. They further surmised that the introduction seemed to have happened in December 2013. However, if Emile died on the 06$^{th}$ of December, then the introduction happened in November. But if he died on the 28$^{th}$ of December (*Zeit Online*), then he certainly was not the index case as the incubation period for toddlers is seven to ten days. As noted above, the fact that his grandmother (S4) died on the 1$^{st}$ of January 2014 implies that she got infected sometime around the first week of December. If Emile died on the 28$^{th}$ of December, then he got infected much later, sometime around the 19$^{th}$ or 20$^{th}$ of December. Notwithstanding, it is also fascinating that some researchers and most journalists contended that a two-year-old first came into contact with the source, especially as they opined that the source was an animal.

Sylvain Baize was honest in admitting that they could not explain how the two-year-old child could have become the first person infected. But rather than let Hollywood writers or overzealous journalists fantasize about the infection of a *suspected* case, a group of researchers led by Mari Saez (postdoctoral researcher at the Institute of Tropical Medicine and International Health) usurped the latter role and had a complete fabrication published in the *EMBO Molecular Medicine Journal* on December 30, 2014. They state that the epidemic stems from a single zoonotic transmission involving Emile Ouamonou, who might have been infected while hunting or playing with insectivorous free-tailed bats in a nearby hollow tree. They seemed to have applied deductive reasoning to arrive at this conclusion. This is because they began by assuming that five propositions were true. The first proposition is that there was a single zoonotic transmission event that was then followed by human (Emile) to human (grandmother, mother, and sister) transmission. They cite the article by Gire et al. published in the *Science* journal on August 28, 2014, to this effect. This article is discussed below since it reports some of the findings of a study that was conducted by six local researchers who suddenly died before it was published.

The second proposition is that hunting and butchering of fruit bats are common activities in Guinea, and children are exposed to bats through hunting. The third proposition is that the two-year-old Emile Ouamonou is Patient Zero. They cite Baize et al. to this effect but do not state that the child is simply the first case that Baize et al. *suspected* had died of the Ebola virus disease due to the recorded prominent symptoms. The fourth proposition is that there was a large hollow tree situated about 50 meters from the home of Emile Ouamonou and close to a path that led to a small river. The villagers told the researchers that children often played in the hollow tree, but it caught fire on March 24, 2014, killing several bats. The fifth proposition is that the consumption of bats by Emile and his family was unlikely to be the source of infection since there was no hunter in the household, and a food item-borne transmission would have affected the adults and children concurrently.

Hence, since children in southern Guinea are exposed to bats through hunting, and there was a hollow tree close to Emile's home that housed bats, they concluded that the two-year-old was infected by a bat in the hollow tree where he had gone hunting.

What is most saddening is that the hypotheses and conditional statements by Saez et al. have repeatedly been reported over the past couple of years as factual. Although an argument may be valid even if one or more of the premises (conditional statements) is false, it cannot be sound. Thus, Saez et al. used fallacious arguments to make an unsound contention. They spent four weeks in southeastern Guinea, including eight days in Meliandou. They captured bats and collected blood and tissue samples but found no evidence of a zoonotic transmission. Moreover, they found no evidence of any decline in the population of remaining large mammals in the area; but ironically found evidence of the increase in the population of chimpanzees. So they insinuated that the bat that allegedly infected Emile Ouamonou did not come into contact with any other person or animal (including fellow bats). This mysterious bat somehow made contact with the two-year-old alone in the hollow tree, 50 meters away from their home, and then did not infect any other animal or person around the village. Other research teams did not find any evidence of a dip in the population of mammals in other areas affected by the disease. Thus, the animal reservoir transmitted the virus to Emile Ouamonou and then vanished without a trace. A more plausible scenario (if we indulge in hypothesizing) would be the consumption of contaminated game by Emile's family that was caught and killed in some other village and brought to Meliandou by a hunter. But then again, there has never been any evidence of any infected animals anywhere in West Africa, even beyond the affected countries. It is only in 1994 that the moderately decayed carcasses of two chimpanzees in the Tai forest in Cote d'Ivoire were found to be aswarm with the Ebola virus. But this was a less virulent strain of the virus, and it is quite distinct from the Zaire Ebola virus that caused the outbreak in 2014. The question that logically follows is whether there was effectively a zoonotic transmission in 2014.

Saez et al. cite the article by Gire et al. to this effect. The latter had noted that although determining phylogeny on the basis of diverse Ebola virus genomes was fraught with difficulties, the phylogenetic comparison that they made suggests that the most recent outbreaks all diverged from a common ancestor at about the same time, sometime in 2004. Hence, each of the last three outbreaks in Africa represents a distinct zoonotic event from the same genetically diverse viral population in the virus' unknown natural reservoir. This does not necessarily imply that the 2014 outbreak in parts of West Africa began with a single zoonotic transmission event but that the Ebola virus responsible for the outbreak came from Central Africa (where there had been a zoonotic transmission) sometime between 2004 and 2014. As such, it is possible that viral specimens may have entered the West African region in a receptacle or frozen blood samples. If the virus came in an animal reservoir as per the official narrative, why did the reservoir not continue to feed the outbreak with new transmissions? As shown above, it is also difficult to contend that this all started with a single zoonotic transmission involving a two-year-old in an isolated area. Also, it is difficult to understand why emphasis has been placed solely on a zoonotic transmission. One of the most important articles on the subject is that written by Kuhn et al. (including Sylvain Baize) and published in *Viruses* journal (6/11) in 2014. The article notes that "Epidemiological and phylogenetic studies indicate that this large [Ebola virus disease] outbreak was caused by a single introduction of one particular ebolavirus, Ebola virus (EBOV), into humans (Homo sapiens) *from an unknown reservoir…*" (Emphasis added). It is interesting that they did not say from an unknown animal reservoir but simply an unknown reservoir. The language is markedly different from that used by Baize et al. a few months earlier in the article in *The New England Journal of Medicine*: "epidemiologic investigation is ongoing to identify the presumed animal source of the outbreak." One then wonders whether Kuhn et al. had a sneaking suspicion that the outbreak was not caused by the introduction of the virus from an animal reservoir.

Sylvain Baize is cited by Denise Grady and Sheri Fink (*The New York Times*) as stating that the consumption of a contaminated fruit is one possibility and "An injection with a contaminated needle is another." This is one of the rare moments where a key researcher in the area has openly considered another possibility of the introduction of the virus into humans. As such, the virus may have been from an animal reservoir or a contaminated needle. The two hypotheses are based on the fact that the study conducted by Baize et al. (*The New*

*England Journal of Medicine*) and most of the subsequent studies had concluded that the epidemiologic links between the cases and the high degree of similarity among the gene sequences suggest a single introduction of the virus into the human population. And this may have happened in December 2013. This implies that sometime in December 2013 one of two things happened: whoever is actually Patient Zero unwittingly consumed a fruit contaminated by the animal reservoir or came in contact with the Ebola Zaire virus that had been released by the animal reservoir; or Patient Zero came into contact with a contaminated needle The latter scenario includes laboratory accidents and human clinical trials. The next two chapters discuss both hypotheses. Nonetheless, it must be noted that in both instances, it is difficult to submit that Emile Ouamonou is Patient Zero or the index case. It is shown above that only in the figment of the overheated imagination of Saez et al. would the first scenario be true because that would imply that the two-year-old Emile was infected by a mysterious animal in the hollow tree about 50 meters away from their house, where he had gone alone to hunt for bats. In the likelihood of the 'reservoir' being a contaminated needle, it may also be difficult to argue that Emile is the index case since that would imply that he was infected in a local clinic or by a sauntering researcher. However, the testimony of the father seems to suggest that the symptoms of the Ebola virus disease (assuming the testimony is accurate) were already prominent before any healthcare professional intervened.

# CHAPTER 4

# Zoonotic Transmission: the Animal Source

Diseases referred to as zoonoses or said to be zoonotic are infectious diseases that originate in animals and naturally cross the species barrier to infect humans. There is a wide array of disease pathogens that can cause familiar and exotic diseases in human hosts. The Ebola virus disease is among the most exotic of these diseases since its distribution across the African, or Asian (The Philippines and China) landscape is almost impossible to delineate with no knowledge of the reservoir. Nonetheless, it remains that animals in the jungle are significant disease reservoirs and the data on the whereabouts of the Ebola virus since 1976 show that only humans and wildlife (bats, chimpanzees, and monkeys) have been infected. It must be noted that bacteria and fungi may also be tissue specific habitats of viruses. Nonetheless, humans and some animals seem to provide specific habitats that allow the Ebola virus to thrive.

Also, given that other viruses similar to the Ebola virus such as the Lassa virus and the Reston virus have been shown to originate from animals, it is only logical to assume that the Ebola virus equally has an animal reservoir. It follows from here that many spillover events have gone unnoticed because they involved a highly pathogenic and virulent strain that quickly killed the human hosts. Thus, one would be hard-pressed to find any article in a peer-reviewed journal that casts doubt on the fact that the Ebola virus disease is a zoonotic disease. The bulk of researchers note that the Ebola virus remains problematic because of the lack of knowledge on how it spreads from its unknown animal reservoir to the human host.

Notwithstanding, there is a plethora of publications on how the virus spreads from one human to another. The poor and sometimes deplorable state of diagnostic and treatment centers in many African countries facilitate the rise in the incidence of such infectious diseases from human to human. The centers often have too few properly trained staff in order to cater effectively to the throng of patients and treat the variety of diseases and dysfunctions that occasionally visit communities like a ghoulish horde to a yearly macabre celebration. Many studies have established that four Ebola virus species have been part of the horde and have caused large outbreaks on the African continent since 1976. The species include the Zaire Ebola virus, Sudan Ebola virus, the Bundibugyo (Uganda) Ebola virus, and the Tai Forest (Cote d'Ivoire) Ebola virus. There is an ongoing debate on the correct nomenclature. However, for the purposes of clarity, the four species are identified here with the names of the countries or places where they first 'appeared.' The same approach has been adopted by many experts in the field.

It is important to note that although the rickety and understaffed treatment centers may sometimes be the proximate cause of an outbreak, they are seldom the source of a point-source outbreak. The Ebola virus disease outbreak in West Africa in 2014 may be categorized as a point-source outbreak because if many of the reported cases in 2014 and 2015 are plotted, the resulting graph will be a bell shaped epidemic curve. The number of infections increased sharply and peaked in the middle of 2014, and then declined sharply. Thus, the treatments centers simply provided the ground wherein the causative agent (Ebola virus) spread within the population to reach new susceptible people visiting at or working in these institutions, but no single treatment center could be said to be the geographical location where the source infected the first cases. Given that infected patients brought the virus to the treatment centers, as was the case with the Kenema General Hospital, it may be contended that there was an independent source that infected the patients and possibly others at a particular geographical location for a short period. However, this independent source may not necessarily be located at a single point in time and place. The independent source may be a migrating animal or human who came into contact with the migrating animal. This is because the Ebola virus disease is an infectious disease that is propagated through diverse contact patterns. Thus, it may also be characterized by propagated outbreaks, and the shape of the epidemic curve may vary according to the activities, customs, and habits of susceptible individuals.

Notwithstanding, the first infected patient who brings the virus to the treatment center may be said to be the 'Patient Zero' because he or she represents a key of the jigsaw puzzle that the medical staff and researchers have to fit together to ascertain the emergence and the life cycle of the causative agent. In such cases, the medical staff and researchers are unable to identify another person who may have transmitted the virus to the first patient who visited the treatment center or another person who may have been infected by the animal reservoir at an earlier date. As such, in this context, 'Patient Zero' is used to describe the first confirmed case and not the first human host. This approach was certainly not adopted in the study of the 2014 outbreak in parts of West Africa because the first confirmed case in Guinea did not help in ascertaining the emergence and life cycle of the Zaire Ebola virus (Makona variant). Nonetheless, it is unfortunate that the researchers did not clearly state and reiterate that the search for 'Patient Zero' (first human host) has so far been futile, and it is ongoing. The failure to be unequivocal has led to gross mischaracterizations and misrepresentations by the sensationalist media.

The above notwithstanding, the point I am trying to make here is that a review of the extant literature on the occurrence of cases of the Ebola virus disease reveals that the source is most likely an animal source, irrespective of whether the outbreak is a point-source outbreak or propagated outbreak. In other words, Patient Zero's infection is most likely to have been caused by contact with an infected animal. An article by Formenty et al. (*The Journal of Infectious Diseases*, 1999) revealed that the Tai Forest (Cote d'Ivoire) Ebola virus was first identified in a chimpanzee that had infected an ethologist performing a necropsy on the animal in the Tai Forest in Cote d'Ivoire (she survived). Also, an article by Miranda et al. (*The Journal of Infectious Diseases*, 1996) revealed that the Reston virus lived and caused disease in non-human pirates in the Philippines. As such, it is only logical to assume that an infected animal was equally the source of the recent emergence of the Ebola virus disease in parts of West Africa. However, although previous studies have established the presence of the Tai Forest (Cote d'Ivoire) Ebola virus in West Africa, the investigation by Baize et al. on the emergence of the disease in Guinea (where the first cases were reported) revealed that the causative agent was the Zaire Ebola virus. Zaire (Democratic Republic of Congo) is in Central or Middle Africa. Baize et al. succinctly describe how this causative agent was detected using conventional Filoviridae-specific RT-PCR assays and performing EBOV-specific real-time RT-PCR.

Kuhn et al. (*Viruses*, 2014) also conducted epidemiological and evolutionary analyses that confirmed that the outbreak of the Ebola virus disease in parts of West Africa in early 2014, as well as the less reported outbreak in the Boende District of the Democratic Republic of Congo in August 2014 (66 cases and 49 deaths recorded), was caused by a single introduction of the Zaire Ebola virus into human populations. They also note that both outbreaks are not related given that they were caused by two new Zaire Ebola virus variants, which they named (based on consensus decisions) "Makona" (West Africa), and "Lomela" (Congo, Central Africa). As regards the 2014 outbreak in parts of West Africa, they cited Baize et al. to the effect that the disease broke out "around Gueckedou, Kissidougou, and Macenta, Guinea" and then spread to at least five countries in the region. This is markedly different from the reports in the media where Baize et al. are cited as stating categorically that the disease broke out in Meliandou in Guinea. Kuhn et al. note further that the outbreak was caused by a single introduction of one particular Ebola virus into humans from an unknown reservoir. Thus, all subsequent cases are derived from one unnamed variant. As noted above, they then named the variant, Makona, after the Makona River flowing close to the triple point of the most affected countries, Guinea, Sierra Leone, and Liberia. It is also worth noting that Kuhn et al. did not say the virus came from an unknown natural or animal reservoir but simply from an unknown reservoir. They also emphasized that the Zaire Ebola virus-Makona was not a strain but a variant in accordance with the definition of 'variant' in standardized filovirus nomenclature. However, they did not state that they had identified any hybrid origin of viral fragments in the variant, implying that there is nothing in their findings to suggest that the new variant may be man-made.

Nonetheless, what is most intriguing here is that prior to the 2014 outbreak, the Ebola virus was not present in Guinea, Liberia and Sierra Leone. It may however equally be stated that prior to the 1976 outbreaks, Sudan and Zaire were not considered areas in which very deadly filoviruses were present. But then again, researchers did not have access to the records of the diagnoses of patients in hospitals and clinics in Sudan and Zaire prior to the 1976 outbreaks. Moreover, the hospitals and clinics in these countries were in a relatively rudimentary stage at the time, and the personnel was certainly not equipped to diagnose most of the deadly diseases caused by filoviruses.

The study conducted by Baize et al. suggests that the introduction seems to have occurred in December 2013, but as noted above, this is unlikely if the first suspected case died in the first week of December 2013. This is because he would then have been infected in November 2013. Also, the researchers are uncertain as to the presumed animal source of the outbreak. They have been unable to identify the reservoir from any of the animals that were in close contact with humans in the region in 2013 and earlier. But then again some researchers have noted that phylogenetic analyses of the full-length sequences have established a separate monophylum or group of the 'Guinean Ebola virus strain' in a sister relationship with other known Ebola virus strains. The contention here is that the so-called Guinean Ebola virus strain had evolved in parallel with the strains from the Democratic Republic of Congo and Gabon (Central Africa) from a common ancestor, and was not introduced in Guinea (West Africa) from Congo or Gabon. Notwithstanding, Kuhn et al. later on established that the causative agent was a variant of the Zaire Ebola virus, not a strain. What they did not say is whether the Zaire Ebola virus-Makona variant was introduced in Guinea or Sierra Leone (West Africa) from Congo or Gabon (Central Africa).

Baize et al. note that it may be important to determine a reliable evolutionary rate of the Ebola virus in nature (using archeological calibration for example). It has been suggested that the Ebola virus that emerged in parts of West Africa in 2014 may be a pre-existing virus that is endemic to this region and has evolved independently from the Zaire Ebola virus into a 'new' variant. The new variant then infected humans when they came in contact with the animal carrying it. This seems to suggest that people in the forested areas all across West and Central Africa are at serious risk. However, it also begs a number of questions: why was there no outbreak prior to December 2013, especially if the source is an animal that has been in contact with humans in the region for some time now? Also, why hasn't there been another outbreak in the same region since early 2014 since the unknown animal reservoir must surely still be interacting with humans there?

Prior to the study conducted by Baize et al., Carroll et al. (*Journal of Virology*, 2013) had estimated that the Ebola virus evolves at about 7 x $10^{-4}$ substitutions per site per year. This in part motivated the argument by Dudas and Rambault (*PLOS Currents*, 2014) that the virus ought to have accumulated in significant amounts of substitutions over the period of almost 38 years since the first recorded outbreak in 1976. Dudas and Rambault then used that to root the Ebola virus tree in order to determine where the 2014 outbreak in parts of West Africa lies. They estimated the phylogeny of the coding sequences using MrBayes, which is a maximum likelihood tree; then they identified the root that gave the best association between genetic divergence and time using the software, Pathogen. They found that there were no suitable outgroup sequences to root the Ebola virus phylogeny, and a temporal rooting gives more consistent results. They then concluded that the outbreak in Guinea was likely caused by a lineage of the Zaire Ebola virus that spread from the latter country or region into Guinea and West Africa in the recent past. They also noted that there is no evidence of a divergent and endemic virus. Moreover, without more diverse sequences from the animal reservoir, it may be difficult to ascertain when the lineage of the Ebola virus from Central Africa was introduced into West Africa. Nonetheless, as mentioned above, subsequent researchers contended that the introduction into humans might have occurred in December 2013. This implies that assuming the transmission was zoonotic, a troop of animals recently left Central Africa aswarm with the Zaire Ebola virus and journeyed over many years for thousands of miles to West Africa, where one of them then transmitted the virus to a human. With regard to that mysterious troop, Baize et al. hypothesized that since potential reservoirs of the Zaire Ebola virus, including the fruit bats of the species *Hypsignathus monstrosus, Epomops franquetti* and *Myonycteris torquata*, are present in many parts of West Africa, it is possible that the virus may have roamed over the region undetected for some time.

As such, unlike reports in the media that cited Baize et al. as stating categorically that the animal reservoir was a fruit bat, it is clear from the above that the link between the 2014 outbreak in parts of West Africa and the fruit bat was based on conjecture. Nonetheless, Baize et al. are not the first researchers to have suggested that the fruit bats were the potential animal reservoirs. These mammals of the order of Chiroptera have for some time now been designated as the most likely culprits.

THE FRUIT BAT: CULPRIT OR SCAPEGOAT?

Whenever a tragedy has befallen humankind, the latter has impetuously cast lots for a scapegoat and sent it into the wilderness of stigmatization and isolation. Without the identification and banishment of the scapegoat, humans remain guarded and are generally too overwrought to perform rational actions. Hence, following the outbreak of the Ebola virus disease in parts of West Africa, researchers combed the dense rainforest of the region in search of the 'scapegoat' that is burdened with the Ebola virus. The identification of the animal would explain how the Zaire Ebola virus, well known in Central or Middle Africa, was able to spread some thousands of miles away. Hence, researchers more than ever felt compelled to find the mysterious animal which was apparently able to transport the deadly virus over thousands of miles without much ado. Researchers from the Institut Pasteur in Lyon, France, who sequenced some of the first samples had expected to find the Tai Forest (Cote d'Ivoire) Ebola virus and were very surprised to find that the causative agent was the Zaire Ebola virus, the deadliest of the four known species. Gretchen Vogel (*Science*, 2014) states that primatologist, Christophe Boesch of the Max Planck Institute for Evolutionary Anthropology in Leipzig, Germany, was frustrated about how the Zaire Ebola virus could have migrated from Central Africa to Guinea (West Africa). However, he suspected that the animal that could have acted as the host or possibly reservoir of the virus and traveled for thousands of miles was the fruit bat. William Karesh of EcoHealth Alliance in New York City is also said to have harbored the same suspicions for a while. This is because some species of the fruit bat of the Central African rainforest had shown evidence of infection without getting sick. A good example is the little collared species, *Myonycteris torquata*, which was found in both Central Africa and West Africa (including Guinea). Thus, following the outbreak in West Africa, researchers sought to ascertain whether the Zaire Ebola virus circulated in bats in the West African forest, especially around the Nzerekore Region in Guinea and the Eastern Province of Sierra Leone, where the first cases were reported. This was the main objective of the study conducted by a team of researchers led by Fabian Leendertz of the Robert Koch Institute, Berlin. They captured and tested several bats and also searched for recent dips in the populations of other animals such as chimpanzees and antelopes, other known hosts of the Ebola virus. They monitored different areas and gathered blow flies that feed on carrion, and analyzed the DNA that persisted in their recent meals. They found nothing. The Ebola virus had once again appeared and disappeared without leaving a trace.

As such, the fruit bat may, after all, be the 'scapegoat' – symbolically burdened with the virus to explain the sudden outbreak in parts of West Africa, thousands of miles away from the home of the Zaire

Ebola virus. This is because prior to the 2014 outbreak in parts of West Africa no case of bat to human transmission had been established. Olival and Hayman (*Viruses* journal, 2014) examined most of the filovirus (Ebola virus and Marburg virus) outbreaks in humans with links to bat exposure between 1967 and 2013. Their findings were to the effect that there have been outbreaks in the Democratic Republic of Congo, Angola, and Uganda in areas that are close to caves known to harbor large bat populations. However, they did not show that these outbreaks were caused by viruses that used the bats in the caves as hosts or reservoirs. Miranda et al. (*The Journal of Infectious Diseases*, 1996) also established epidemiological links between bats and filoviruses following multiple transmission events in mines in Kenya but did not show that any outbreaks were actually caused by viruses that used the bats in the mines as hosts or reservoirs. Equally, Peterson et al. (*Emerging Infectious Diseases*, 2004) and Peterson (*Emerging Infectious Diseases*, 2006) used ecological niche models to provide regional views on the distribution of the Ebola and Marburg viruses and suggested that bats, mice, and shrew species may be sources of the infection. They did not establish the validity of the hypothesis by the presentation of evidence. Also, Swanepoel et al. (*Emerging Infectious Diseases*, 2007) examined several potential hosts of the Marburg virus in a mine in the Democratic Republic of Congo associated with an outbreak between 1998 and 2000. They found that although the bats were infected, they had developed an antibody to the virus and survived the infection. This corresponds with a previous study conducted by Leroy et al. (*Nature*, 2005) which showed that three fruit bat species were reservoirs of Ebola virus RNA and had developed anti-Ebola virus antibodies.

In light of the above, it may be submitted that despite the cogent theoretical link between human infection and bat exposure, there is no evidence to confirm this. Researchers have for example observed that bats in the Ugandan caves contracted and replicated the Marburg virus especially during birthing season, and most human cases were diagnosed during birthing season as well, but the researchers could not find any evidence that the miners and tourists in the area who had been diagnosed with Marburg fever had actually been infected by the bats in the caves. In the same vein, the link between the 2014 outbreak of the Ebola virus disease in parts of West Africa and bat exposure is still very conjectural. No researcher has so far been able to identify the fruit bat that traversed the vast distance from Central Africa to West Africa with the Zaire Ebola virus in its system. Also, if such fruit bats are the reservoirs, then it may be difficult to explain why the outbreak is not much wider given that many people in the forest area of West Africa eat fruit bats. The interactions between humans and fruit bats across the region are therefore too frequent to justify a single spillover event. There is good reason to contend that the special emphasis on bats is due to the fact that the interactions between humans and wildlife create an environment that is conducive to spillover events, and humans in the affected countries interact with bats more than any other animal in the rainforest. Nonetheless, if the virus has been circulating in bats in the area for any reasonable period, it is likely that there would have been many more outbreaks in different regions. This is because, as mentioned above, the migratory fruit bats are eaten in many different West African countries. The locals also often come into contact with the urine and feces of these bats, and the latter sometimes use the houses of humans as roosting places.

It is true that it has been pointed out that there may have been previous spillover events that went unnoticed because humans are generally a dead end. However, it is unlikely that in this day and age, scores of humans in a village could die from a mysterious illness without anyone raising an alarm. A cross-section of West Africans work in urban or semi-urban areas or have family working there. Thus, it is improbable that those in urban or semi-urban areas would not be alerted about an outbreak of a deadly disease in a rural area or even in the hinterlands. Most clans or large families have a head (usually the most resourceful person) living in an urban area, and whenever members of the clan or large family in the hinterlands are very afflicted, they flock to the city and notify the head who has a moral obligation to resolve problems faced by the clan or family.

It must also be noted that antelopes and chimpanzees may also act as intermediaries in the transmission of the Ebola virus from bats to humans, given that humans in these areas eat antelopes and chimpanzees as well. Antelopes are prized game. However, this transmission chain is improbable since Fabian Leendertz revealed that they did not stumble across any dead animals, and there were no obvious epidemics among animals that might have acted as intermediaries. Also, as noted above, Saez et al. found evidence of the increase in the population of chimpanzees. The Tai Forest (Cote d'Ivoire) Ebola virus was discovered because it left dead chimpanzees in its wake. Thus, it is unlikely that the Ebola virus disease caused by the Zaire Ebola virus may have burned itself out in West Africa with antelopes and chimpanzees.

In light of the above, one may wonder whether the bat is the culprit or simply the animal chosen by lot as the scapegoat. It has certainly not been symbolically burdened with the Ebola virus given that there is evidence that it is a reservoir of the virus. However, it has been symbolically burdened with the Zaire Ebola virus-Makona variant that caused the 2014 outbreak in parts of West Africa. This may be seen in several reports published by the mainstream media in North America and Western Europe since the outbreak. In fact, a few months after the outbreak it was an anecdote of sorts; a year after, it was reported as part of the 'official' narrative. It is uncertain why many of the researchers who have clearly concluded that the link between the 2014 outbreak and the fruit bat is based on conjecture, for the time being, have been largely unconcerned about media reports citing them as stating categorically that the fruit bat is the culprit. I set out to determine why the media had chosen to report the story about a fruit bat infecting a two-year-old in Meliandou as factual, and also why the researchers cited as the source of the story were unconcerned about the misrepresentation. I then wrote to two of the most cited news outlets in the United Kingdom that had covered the 2014 outbreak in West Africa extensively and given the impression that they were relaying information from researchers on the ground.

## THE GUARDIAN

On Saturday, August 23, 2014, *The Guardian* published an article titled: "Ebola: Research Team Says Migrating Fruit Bats Responsible for Outbreak." It was written by John Vidal. The first paragraph reads as follows:

"The largest-ever outbreak of Ebola was triggered by a toddler's chance contact with a single infected bat, a team of international researchers will reveal, after a major investigation of the origins of the deadly disease now ravaging Guinea, Liberia, Ivory Coast and Nigeria."

By the time I began writing this book, at the end of 2014, the disease "ravaging" Nigeria had been effectively contained, and only one case was reported in Ivory Coast throughout the crisis. The team of international researchers is the aforementioned team led by Fabian Leendertz of the Robert Koch Institute which is still working on the link between human infection and bat exposure, discussed extensively by previous researchers, some of whom are cited above. *The Guardian* nonetheless cites Fabian Leendertz as stating that the straw-colored fruit bat had probably conveyed the Zaire Ebola virus. However, the article does not state that Fabian Leendertz justified the claim with evidence of positive tests of the bats his team had captured and tested. Instead, it notes that the researcher justified the claim with another claim that the fruit bat was the potential reservoir because these mammals are known to migrate across long distances and may be found in large colonies near cities and forests. This is a fallacy of assumptions, which was wrongly imputed to the researcher. The article then moved to the story of the putative Patient Zero, the 2-year old boy who allegedly caught the disease during a chance encounter with an infected bat in Meliandou. As noted several times above, this theory is based on Baize et al.'s postulate published in the *The New England Journal of Medicine* shortly after the outbreak. However, the theory is presented in the article as part of Fabian Leendertz's team's findings.

## THE DAILY MAIL

On Sunday, August 24, 2014, *The Daily Mail* published an article by Paul Donnelley titled:

"Ebola outbreak sweeping West Africa started with two-year-old boy infected by a fruit bat, say researchers."

Paul Donnelley equally gives the impression that his source is the "17-strong team of European and African tropical disease researchers, ecologists and anthropologists ....led by Fabian Leendertz ..." The latter is quoted to have said that an infected straw-colored fruit bat brought the disease to Guinea. Then the reader is allowed to presume that it is the same source that revealed that the straw-colored fruit bat bit a two-year-old boy, and the latter passed the infection on to his mother, and both were dead within a week. The disease was then spread to the community by mourners who came to the funeral. Later on in the article, Fabian Leendertz is quoted as implying that the straw-colored fruit bat may have brought the disease to Guinea because they are known to travel long distances and usually settle in forests near cities. Thus, "an individual bat or colony [may have] migrated all the way from Congo or Gabon to West Africa." As noted above, the possibility of bat to human transmission is quite strong since villagers in Guinea, Sierra Leone, and Liberia regularly catch, kill, and eat bats. However, Paul Donnelley does not ponder the question of why other infected bats have not transmitted the virus to other humans and caused other spillover events and outbreaks in other West African countries. In the case of the Machupo virus that infected humans in Bolivia in 1963, it was easy to establish such a pattern given that the native mice that were identified as the reservoir of the virus had carried the virus into several dwellings and granaries. Thus, the outbreak was ended when the mice were trapped out. In the case of the Ebola virus disease in West Africa, if the reservoir host was an animal (bat, non-human primate or mouse), the person least likely to be the first infected through this chain is a two-year-old; surely the adults who kill and cook dozens of bats each day would have been infected first. Hence, although Fabian Leendertz clearly stated that the premise was yet to be proved, it was presented as a fact.

On the 6th of November 2014, I sent the following email to John Vidal of *The Guardian*:

> *Dear John Vidal,*
>
> *I am currently conducting a study on media reports on the recent outbreak of Ebola in West Africa.*
>
> *You published an article in **The Guardian on Saturday August 23rd, 2014** with the title:*
>
> ***Ebola: Research Team Says Migrating Fruit Bats Responsible for Outbreak***
>
> *However, the research team led by Fabian Leendertz (which you cite as source) never claimed that the fruit bats were*

*responsible - they are working on that supposition but it has not been proved.*

*Moreover, you also state as follows:*

*"The largest-ever outbreak of Ebola was triggered by a toddler's chance contact with a single infected bat."*

*Also, this is yet to be established and the reference to a deceased two-year-old as patient zero is not based on the study conducted by Fabian Leendertz's team but on the epidemiologic look-back investigation of the transmission chains performed by a team led by Sylvain Baize. Thus, the two-year-old is simply the first recorded case according to hospital documentations and interviews with affected families as interpreted by Sylvain Baize's team.*

*Thus, it may be important to know why you were categorical about the source of the outbreak in your article when this is far from being established. Also, it is uncertain why you state that the two-year-old (identified by Sylvain Baize's team and who may even have died from some other disease) was infected by a bat.*

*Thank you so much in advance for your response*

*Kind regards,*
*Constantine Nana*

John Vidal did not reply.

I retrieved the email sent to John Vidal, replaced his name with Paul Donnelley, and sent the email to the latter and still await his response. The silence of these men of the media is disconcerting but not unexpected since it is stereotypical of the 'Western' media that would sometimes heartily alter information and evidence in order to oblige the macabre romanticism of poverty porn.

On the 6th of November 2014, I sent this message to Fabian Leendertz:

*Dear Dr. Leendertz,*

*I am currently conducting a study on media reports on the recent outbreak of Ebola in West Africa. You are cited in several of the reports because of the work done by your team in Meliandou (Gueckedou). However, I would like to know why you allow these papers to cite you as stating that the source of Ebola virus (EBOV) in Guinea is the straw-colored fruit bat when this has not been established? Also, the papers give the impression that you found the two-year-old that was first infected by the fruit bat. Lastly, although the fruit bats are the most likely reservoirs, if none of the bats you caught and tested in Guinea had the virus, is it possible that the source of the outbreak may not be an animal?*

*Thank you so much in advance for your answers,*
*Constantine*

On the 7th of November 2014, Fabian Leendertz's reply came in. He stated categorically that the statement by *The Guardian* journalist (John Vidal) regarding the straw-colored fruit bat "was made up" by the journalist. He noted further that the supposed Patient Zero was described in the paper by Baize et al. and not by his team. However, for some unknown reason, the esteemed researcher decided to keep me in suspense by stating that he did not say that his team had not found the virus in the affected region, and this would be known when their findings are published. Then he asked me to explain the surmise regarding the source of the outbreak not being an animal.

Although I was most grateful for Fabian Leendertz's candid response, I did not answer the question he posed because I was still straining to excogitate upon a source other than an animal. Hence, at the time my response would only have sounded like the pompous and ill-founded claim of a conceited blogger. As shown above, the Internet is awash with baseless claims about other sources of the outbreak. Thus, it is wise to consider the possibility of a non-animal source very carefully before making any claim, even when the researchers on the ground are still vacillating between suppositions. Non-animal sources are considered in the next chapter. What is important to note here is that the Zaire Ebola virus was brought to the treatment centers in West Africa by one or many infected patients who had been infected by an independent source at a specific geographical location for a given period. However, this independent source was not necessarily located at a single point in time and place given that the Ebola virus disease is an infectious disease that is propagated through diverse contact patterns. Despite the unequivocal media reports, the search for that independent source continues. The data of the study conducted by Fabian Leendertz's team has since been published, and they did not find the virus in any of the blood and tissue samples collected. Like previous researchers after previous outbreaks, they had ransacked the African forest for the Ebola virus in vain. The virus had once again appeared and disappeared, together with its mysterious reservoir. The reservoir is most likely an animal (the fruit bat, antelope, or chimpanzee or maybe even a human), but as will be shown in the next chapter, the claim about a non-animal source is not altogether extraordinary.

# CHAPTER 5

# The Theory of the 'Contaminated Needle'

There is consensus on the fact that the 2014 Ebola virus disease epidemic in parts of West Africa stemmed from a single transmission of the virus to the index case, without further exposure of any human to the host or reservoir. This implies that after the first transmission of the virus from the source, no other human has come into contact with that source. This screams laboratory accident or human clinical trial to the cynic. This is because unless Patient Zero happened upon a contaminated needle that had dropped from the heavens, it is difficult to ascertain how an outbreak starts with a single introduction of the virus only to Patient Zero, and no other persons or animals are exposed to the source; and there is no trace of the source afterwards.

The Zaire Ebola virus, the species that ran amok in West Africa, has caused epidemics in the past with case fatality rates of up to 90%. It is therefore considered a Biosafety Level 4 agent and experiments with the virus ought to be performed in a Biosafety Level 4 laboratory. This is an enclosed laboratory facility with the highest level of biocontainment precautions required to work with dangerous and deadly agents. Additional safety measures must be implemented because Biosafety Level 4 agents pose a very high individual risk of infection. A pathogen is also considered a Biosafety Level 4 agent because it may cause very severe to fatal disease in humans, and no vaccine or treatments are available. It is, therefore, mandatory that positive pressure personnel suits are used, as well as a separate air supply. Also, the air and water supply going to and coming from the facility are decontaminated to minimize accidental releases. Equally, there are safety precautions designed to destroy the agents at the entrance and exit of the laboratory, including a vacuum room, multiple showers, and an ultraviolet light room. Coupled with the fact that the users of the laboratory are for the most part people with expert knowledge, they are given specific training in handling dangerous and infectious agents and are supervised by other experienced experts.

Despite these safety measures, Gunther et al., in an article published in 2011 in *The Journal of Infectious Diseases* on the management of a laboratory accident with the Ebola virus in the Biosafety Level 4 laboratory at the Bernhard Nocht Institute for Tropical Medicine in Germany, note that there have been three documented laboratory accidents with the Ebola virus. As will be shown below, there have been more. The first accident reported by Gunther et al. occurred in 1976 at the Microbiological Research Establishment in Porton Down near Stonehenge in the United Kingdom. David Quammen in his book *Ebola: The Natural and Human History of A Deadly Virus*, describes the research center as "a discreetly expert institution" and "an experiment station for the development of chemical weapons such as mustard gas." He notes further that during the Second World War, researchers at the Institute conducted studies on biological weapons derived from anthrax and botulin bacteria. He then claims that the focus of the researchers has since shifted to countermeasures against biological and chemical weapons. It is, however, uncertain whether a fine line may be drawn between research on weaponizing pathogens and research on countermeasures against weaponized pathogens. Certainly, in both instances the pathogens have to be weaponized, either hypothetically or in actuality. This is because when conducting research on countermeasures against weaponized pathogens, the countermeasures are certainly devised to negate an actual or hypothetically weaponized pathogen. However, in an article published by Amy Shurtleff et al. in the *Viruses* journal (December 19, 2012), it is noted that there are strict regulations on research conducted in Biosafety Level 4 laboratories that limit the size of projects and the number of collaborations. The researchers are screened and monitored continuously. They are required to comply with time limits and must test and assess new therapeutics and vaccines under conditions approved by the FDA. Thus, researchers who seek to modify or weaponize pathogens have more leeway in testing and assessing their findings.

Notwithstanding, the accident in Porton Down was not related to research on countermeasures or attempts at weaponizing the Ebola virus. At the time, the virus was not known to the researchers at the Institute. It did not even have a name. It had arrived in deeply frozen blood samples from patients in Sudan, and the researchers were asked to identify the agent that was killing people in Sudanese villages with remarkable swiftness and efficiency. In the course of carrying out the assignment, one of the researchers, Geoffrey Platt, pierced his thumb through a protective rubber glove while trying to inject the homogenized liver of an infected guinea pig into another test animal. Although there was no bleeding, Platt was alarmed because almost half of the infected patients in Sudan had succumbed to the disease in a matter of weeks. One can therefore only imagine his apprehension at the fact that the contaminated needle had effectively punctured his thumb, although it was the slightest of punctures. This would later reveal to other researchers how potent the Ebola virus can be. Exposure to an extremely small dose was enough to cause infection and potentially kill the patient. The circumstances surrounding this case were presented in an article by Edmond et al. published in the *British Medical Journal* in 1977. They noted that Platt became ill six days after exposure. The first symptoms were nausea, exhaustion, and abdominal pain. At the high-security infectious diseases unit at the Coppetts Wood Hospital near London, he was administered interferon and blood serum from Sudanese patients who had 'mysteriously' recovered from the disease. However, four days later his immune system was dysfunctional. He had diarrhea and vomited, and had fungal growth in his throat. He was given more borrowed antibodies. Two days later, the vomiting and diarrhea inexplicably ceased, and the virus suddenly vanished from his blood, urine, and feces (except his semen).

Some 28 years later, the most controversial of the reported accidents occurred in a Biosafety Level 4 laboratory at the Vektor Research Institute of Molecular Biology near Novosibirsk in Russia. This institute is the only repository of the deadly smallpox virus in the world, apart from the Centers for Disease Control and Prevention in Atlanta. A note published in the *Science* journal on May 28, 2004, states that the accident involved an Ebola researcher called Antonina Presnyakova who pricked her hand with a contaminated needle. She had drawn blood from an infected guinea pig with a syringe. A report from the *Itar-Tass News* agency published on May 22, 2004, on the ProMED-mail website said: "[her] hand just slipped and she jabbed herself."

It is stated further that she developed the prominent symptoms about one week later and died on May 19, 2004, exactly two weeks after infection. Given that the WHO does not require research centers to report accidents involving the Ebola virus unless the accidents pose a threat to the public, it is alleged that the Vektor Research Institute only reported the incident and sought help from the WHO two days before Antonina passed on. It is uncertain whether her life would have been saved if the Vektor Research Institute had contacted the WHO sooner. Nonetheless, due to the alleged delay, other researchers across the world were not able to provide prompt advice that may have saved her life. At the time, the Vektor Research Institute claimed it did all that could be done and would publish a report following an internal inquiry. The *Itar-Tass* report also claimed that she was isolated in a special unit and treated in consultation with experts from the Health Ministry, including Russian healthcare professionals who had treated Ebola patients in Africa.

An article by Judith Miller published in *The New York Times* on May 25, 2004, noted that the Biosafety Level 4 laboratory at the Vektor Research Institute was a former biological weapons laboratory that was specialized in weaponizing deadly viruses. The institute then received funding from the United States to help convert their research programs to peaceful research programs. Organizations from the United States apparently spent close to $10 million to this effect. Antibody Systems Inc, a US-based producer of biological materials for research, for example, spent more than $150,000 over five years on joint studies on Ebola at the Vektor Research Institute. Nonetheless, Antonina was not part of the program sponsored by Antibody Systems, and it is uncertain who was financing her research given that neither the nature nor goal of the research was disclosed. The non-disclosure of the nature of the research and the reluctance to inform the WHO (as well as the laboratory directors at the Institute, according to *The New York Times*) about the accident certainly raise many unsettling questions. Many researchers in the United States opposed the allocation of resources to the Russian research institute on the grounds that it was uncertain whether Russian researchers had ceased carrying out studies aimed at weaponizing deadly viruses. In the 1990s, many offensive research programs (or the weaponizing of viruses) were officially ended. Many assembly lines were dismantled, and some facilities became pharmaceutical plants. However, some commentators such as Ken Alibek and Stephen Handelman (*Biohazard: The Chilling True Story of the Largest Covert Biological Weapons Program in the World*) argued that Russia still treasured its biological warfare infrastructure. This is because facilities that had been transformed into pharmaceutical plants were still sealed off from the public and were never opened to foreign inspection.

Nonetheless, Natalia Skultetskaya, the spokesperson of the Vektor Research Institute, is quoted in an article in the *Sydney Morning Herald* (May 25, 2004) as stating that the WHO and Russian Ministry of Health were informed of the accident in the Institute's Biosafety Level 4 laboratory in a timely manner. She also intimated that there had been previous laboratory accidents involving filoviruses. In 1988, a researcher accidentally contracted the Marburg virus and died. In 1996, a researcher at the Defense Ministry's Virology Center in Sergiyey Posad (near Moscow) accidentally contracted the Ebola virus and died. Natalia Skultetskaya then noted that like the two previous researchers, Antonina was conducting studies on the Ebola and Marburg viruses with the goal of developing a vaccine. She said progress had been made. However, she did not mention any publications (past or future) of the findings to demonstrate the progress.

Interestingly, an article by Mark Franchetti published on the website of *The Australian* on October 26, 2014, provides a different version. Mark Franchetti's sources include an unnamed former Russian bioweapons researcher and *The Washington Post*. He claims that the accident that occurred in 1996 at the Defense Ministry's Virology Center in Sergiyey Posad was related to a secret biological weapons program set up by the Soviet Union. He says Nadezhda Makovetskaya, a female laboratory technician, pricked herself with a contaminated needle as she drew blood from a horse that had been infected. She died a few days later and was buried with a "sack filled with calcium hypochlorite." He then claims (without any evidence) that Antonina had equally been conducting bioweapons research when she was infected, and Russian researchers until a few years ago (the article was published in 2014) still conducted biological weapons research by cultivating microbes as weapons of war. He further intimates that the research conducted by Antonina sought to assess the potential of the Ebola virus as a biological weapon, and it involved manipulating the genetic coding of the virus. However, Russian researchers had subsequently concluded that the virus was not well suited for biowarfare. He then insinuates that this is what prompted the Russian government to announce that researchers at the Vektor Research Institute and the Defense Ministry's Virology Center had developed experimental vaccines. It is important to point out that Mark Franchetti also said Russian officials had accused the United States of hypocrisy on the grounds that researchers in the United States have also been conducting offensive research, including the weaponizing of pathogens such as the Ebola virus. As shown in Chapter 2, studies that sought to enhance the response to public health and bioterrorism threats posed by the deadly filoviruses were unusually connected to the research on Lassa fever in West Africa shortly before the outbreak of the Ebola virus disease in 2014. Extensive studies on biological threats have equally been undertaken by the United States Army Medical Research Institute of Infectious Diseases (USAMRIID) for many decades. This led to an accident in a laboratory in the United States in 2004.

Thus, in the same year in which a fatal laboratory accident occurred in a Biosafety Level 4 laboratory at the Vektor Research Institute in Russia, a virologist working in the Biosafety Level 4 laboratory at the USAMRIID was almost infected with blood from a mouse laden with a *mouse-adapted variant* of the Zaire Ebola virus. Emphasis is placed on *mouse-adapted variant* here because this was a man-made variant and is further evidence that the Zaire Ebola virus was being constantly modified in order to determine how it would adapt to different environments. The circumstances surrounding the accident at the USAMRIID laboratory were presented in an article by Kortepeter et al. that was published in the *Emerging Infectious Diseases Journal* in 2008. The virologist was working with mice that had been infected with the virus two days before the accident. It is stated that he followed the standard procedure and held the mice intraperitoneally while injecting them with an immune globulin concoction. However, he used the same hypodermic syringe on all the mice. So, when he began injecting the fifth mouse with the syringe, it kicked and shoved the needle into his left hand. The needle pierced the hand through the gloves. His first reaction was to squeeze the laceration to force the extravasation of blood. The injured site was then irrigated with a liter of sterile water, and povidone-iodine was rubbed against it for about ten minutes. Lastly, the blue suit was decontaminated in the chemical shower.

Despite the fact that there were most likely low levels of virus on the needle and the potential for infection was largely reduced by the needle piercing through the gloves, the executive staff at the USAMRIID quarantined the virologist. He was then monitored for routine signs, and regular assessments were performed by a physician. Kortepeter et al. noted that the executive staff informed local public health authorities and consulted several hemorrhagic fever experts on potential treatments. It was agreed that there was no safe treatment that was readily available. However, they considered administering the recombinant nematode protein (rNAPc2) and antisense oligomers if the virologist showed evidence of infection. Equally, the five mice that had been infected with the mouse-adapted variant of the virus did not confirm viremia at the time of the laboratory accident. Nonetheless, the virologist never became ill or seroconvert, and was released after 21 days.

This case report contrasts with that of the accident that occurred in the Biosafety Level 4 laboratory at the Vektor Research Institute in

Russia; albeit the case reports of the incident in Russia that I analyzed are from Western journals and media articles. Notwithstanding, the executive staff of USAMRIID are said to have immediately reported the incident to the local public health authorities and consulted with filovirus experts across the world on potential treatments. This may be contrasted with the Vektor Research Institute's alleged reporting of the incident and seeking help from the WHO more than one week after the laboratory accident. The American media and some American researchers had a sneaking suspicion that the Russians were seeking to weaponize the Ebola virus. This was partly based on the alleged testimony of former Russian bioweapons researchers such as the unnamed researcher that provided information to Mark Franchetti of *The Australian*. Nonetheless, there is nothing to suggest that the American researchers were not equally seeking to weaponize the pathogen. After all, the researchers were using a man-made variant of the Ebola virus and the study was being conducted in a laboratory owned and managed by the United States Army.

As noted above, the circumstances surrounding the laboratory accident at the Bernhard Nocht Institute in Germany were presented by Gunther et al. in an article published in 2011 in *The Journal of Infectious Diseases*. The facts are very similar to the accident at the Biosafety Level 4 laboratory at the USAMRIID. However, the accident in Germany happened about five years later. It involved a virologist injecting concentrated culture supernatant (containing the Zaire Ebola virus) into mice for immunization. When the virologist tried to recap the needle, it pierced through the cap and all three gloves and punctured his skin. Tests conducted after the accident revealed that the Ebola virus retains its infectivity after mixing with Freund's adjuvant. The virologist's wound was disinfected upon leaving the laboratory. Then he was examined by an infectious disease specialist at the University Medical Center in Hamburg. On the same day, a teleconference was held with researchers in the United States and

Canada to discuss potential treatments. After the teleconference, a vaccine known as VSVΔG/ZEBOVGP was shipped to Hamburg, Germany from Winnipeg, Canada; and an emergency clearance from customs was obtained. The following day, another teleconference was held with several filovirus researchers from American and Canadian institutions, including the USAMRIID and the University of Texas Medical Branch. The researchers discussed the potential administration of rNAPc2, the recombinant human activated protein C, and experimental vaccines. They, however, recommended post-exposure vaccination with live-attenuated recombinant vesicular stomatitis virus (recVSV) because it showed a good safety profile in nonhuman primates (NHPs). They also advised that if it was confirmed that the virologist was infected with the Ebola virus, then rNAPc2 should be administered because it is an inhibitor of tissue factor which has demonstrated some therapeutic potential in NHPs infected with the virus. Two days after the incident, a biopharmaceutical company based in Colorado, ARCA Biopharma, released a batch of rNAPc2, and Tekmira Pharmaceuticals (discussed above) provided lipid-nonparticle-encapsulated short interfering RNAs (siRNAs) adapted to target the Ebola virus. Thi et al. in an article published in May 2015 in the *Nature* journal note that siRNAs have been able to provide a 100% protection to rhesus monkeys against the Ebola virus when the treatment began three days after exposure.

The VSVΔG/ZEBOVGP vaccine from Canada was administered to the virologist in Germany two days after exposure. The next day the patient developed fever and myalgia, but these symptoms were not treated given that it was uncertain whether this was a reaction to the vaccine or the onset of the Ebola hemorrhagic fever. However, that evening the patient's temperature returned to normal. He was monitored for the ensuing days as no signs or symptoms developed, and other laboratory parameters remained normal. 14 days after exposure, the patient was transferred to the regular infectious disease ward and discharged from the hospital seven days later.

Gunther et al. in the article published in 2011 in *The Journal of Infectious Diseases* note that the management of this accidental exposure to the Ebola virus by the Bernhard Nocht Institute in Germany has been very helpful because of the Institute's timely communication with the research community. This may once again be contrasted with the operational plan allegedly adopted by the Vektor Research Institute that involved reporting the incident and seeking help from the WHO more than one week after the laboratory accident. Concerning the accident in the laboratory at the Bernhard Nocht Institute, the teleconferences and extensive email communications within a few hours of exposure constituted unique brainstorming sessions. The researchers and physicians involved were able to exchange unpublished findings and investigational vaccines, and drugs were tested without adhering to rigid bureaucratic rules and procedures. Gunther et al. state that the Bernhard Nocht Institute adopted an ad hoc procedure rather than a defined operational plan for the management of accidental exposure in laboratories, and the virologists and clinicians at the Institute knew about the different experimental treatment options. The practicality of the procedure adopted by the Bernhard Nocht Institute cannot be questioned given the urgency of the situation. However, the management of this exposure may be contrasted sharply with that of the infection by Sierra Leone's 'Ebola Doctor' Sheikh Umar Khan during the 2014 outbreak. The bizarre procedure adopted and decisions that were taken, which more or less ensured that Sheikh Umar Khan died, would baffle any informed observer whatsoever. It is amazing how they succeeded in perplexing a situation so plain in itself. This is discussed below.

The above cases demonstrate that research on the Ebola virus is fraught with peril even in enclosed laboratory facilities that are designed for work with very dangerous and exotic pathogens. The researchers all had specific and comprehensive training in dealing with extremely hazardous infectious agents and understood the containment functions of the practices, but they got exposed to the virus. One can only imagine how far more dangerous it is to work with the Ebola virus in a laboratory that is not suitable for such work, or even in a laboratory with a low level of containment designed for work involving agents of only moderate potential hazard to the researchers and the environment. If the virus, for example, had arrived in deep-frozen blood samples at the Biosafety Level 2 laboratory of the Lassa Fever Ward of the Kenema Government Hospital, any study conducted on the virus there would have increased the risk of exposure to exponential levels. The fact that the researchers are fully trained in handling extremely hazardous pathogens is no guarantee that there won't be any accident as shown above. There were Ebola virus disease experts in The Consortium's research team that conducted studies on Lassa fever in Sierra Leone, Liberia, and Nigeria prior to the Ebola outbreak in 2014. It is shown above that this team equally conducted studies on the most potent filovirus, the Ebola virus. Thus, they could very well have imported samples containing the Zaire Ebola virus into Sierra Leone or Guinea and then by pure mischance come in contact with the virus.

This would not be the first time that researchers have announced that they are studying one disease when in fact they are conducting a combined study (involving the Ebola virus). Many reasons (mischief aside) may explain this strategy: lack of funding, lack of support from the hierarchy, sensitiveness of the study, etc. Some members of the International Commission that was set up to combat the Ebola virus disease in Zaire in 1976 still sought to identify the reservoir and any antibodies in the reservoir's blood after they had successfully contained the disease in the Bumba area. Thus, although their mission was complete, they still had the burning desire to identify the source of the virus and determine how spillover took place. Unable to obtain funding to this effect, they submitted a proposal for research on monkeypox and conducted a combined study on both monkeypox

and Ebola. They collected samples from 117 species in the previous
Ebola hotspot; the animals were mostly trapped or hunted by the local
villagers in exchange for monetary rewards offered by the researchers.
The samples included blood and bits of liver, kidney, and spleen of the
animals. Johnson et al. noted in an article subsequently published in
*The Journal of Infectious Diseases* that the covert study was futile as the
researchers found no evidence of Ebola virus infection.

It must be pointed out that the samples collected by these researchers
were not handled in a Biosafety Level 4 laboratory, implying that
the risk of exposure to the Zaire Ebola virus was extremely high.
The researchers surely knew of the risk only so well but went ahead
with the study. Fortunately for the locals and unfortunately for
unethical research, they did not find any trace of the Ebola virus
that had previously ravaged villages in the Bumba area of Zaire.
Nonetheless, if they had found the virus and it then escaped and
caused another outbreak, it is hard to believe that the researchers
would have admitted that the outbreak was caused by exposure to
the virus during a covert study. The unaffected villagers and their
appetite for game seems a ready-made explanation for such events.
After all, the animals tested were trapped or hunted (and most likely
eaten afterward) by the local villagers.

It has also been established that researchers have been exposed to
the Ebola virus in the wild. Formenty et al. in a paper published
in *The Journal of Infectious Diseases* (1999) stated that an ethologist
was infected while examining the body of a dead wild chimpanzee.
This happened in November 1994 in Cote d'Ivoire and marked
the first recorded occurrence of the Ebola virus in West Africa.
The ethologist was inadvertently exposed to a less potent strain of
the Ebola virus (the Tai Forest Ebola virus or Cote d'Ivoire Ebola
virus). She was examining one of the several dead chimpanzees
found in the jungle. Surprisingly, this case was not well documented,

despite the experience and training of the researchers involved. No tests for hemorrhagic fever (Lassa fever or Ebola virus disease) were conducted because the patient did not bleed. The Ebola virus was only detected by immunohistochemistry in the organs of the chimpanzee that had been examined. Thus, this case is one of the stranger ones in the Ebola compendium. It is likely that the ethologist was exposed because she had worn household gloves while the two other researchers who also conducted necropsies on the wild chimpanzees wore latex examination gloves. None of them wore masks or gowns. Hence, the two other researchers were very lucky. They tested negative because no droplets were projected onto their faces. But then again, they had direct face-to-face contact with their infected colleague before the onset of her illness and during her illness. Also lucky were the four laboratory technicians who handled the chimpanzee's organs, as well the 18 persons who had had direct contact with the patient in Cote d'Ivoire, and 52 persons in Switzerland. Nonetheless, the questions about where this "strain" of the Ebola virus came from and how it simply vanished into thin air remain unanswered. However, what is most puzzling is that twenty years later, when the Ebola virus re-emerged in West Africa, it was not as the mysterious Tai Forest (Cote d'Ivoire) Ebola virus but as the more potent Zaire Ebola virus.

What is clear from the above is that if the 18 contact persons in Cote d'Ivoire had become exposed to the Tai Forest (Cote d'Ivoire) Ebola virus, it would have been the onset of an Ebola virus disease outbreak. The transmission chain would have been from the mysterious chimpanzees to the researcher, to the local researchers and assistants, and then the friends and families of the latter. One may then deduce that this may equally have been the case with the Ebola virus disease outbreak in parts of West Africa in 2014. However, if this was the case, then, it is likely that the infection or death of one of the researchers (may be a member of The Consortium) would have been reported shortly before the outbreak or early on during the epidemic. But then again, some local researchers working with The Consortium reportedly got infected during the epidemic and died in the month of July, six or seven months after the outbreak.

So what if the person that was exposed was a low-level local researcher or laboratory assistant at the Biosafety Level 2 laboratory of the Lassa Fever Ward of Kenema Government Hospital? Local researchers or assistants are quite dependable, and due to the horrendously low levels of accountability in African institutions, no one would ask probing and clarifying questions about the nature and cause of the local researchers' illness. The senior local researchers at the Lassa Fever Ward would have been in the best position to affirm this scenario. However, the senior local researchers at the Lassa Fever Ward who worked with The Consortium are unfortunately all dead; killed by the Ebola virus, as well as the inexplicable decision of their foreign colleagues not to administer any of the available experimental treatments to them. The decision was made despite the fact these experimental treatments had proved effective in non-human clinical trials and were duly considered in previous cases of the infection of researchers in Germany and the United States as shown above. Also, the experimental treatments were administered to Western researchers and health workers who got infected during the epidemic in West Africa. Notwithstanding, it goes without saying that the above scenario is simply an instance of inferring an unknown from another unknown; a conjecture formed on the basis of suspicion and intrigue. Such a conjecture/hypothesis would no doubt be easily slashed with Occam's razor because it contains more assumptions than the accepted theory that the outbreak was caused by a villager's chance encounter with an infected animal, and the animal may have been the reservoir or another host in the chain. Nonetheless, as noted above, Occam's razor is not an irrefutable principle of logic, and it is sometimes reasonable to make existential statements or observations that are based on an alternative and plausible explanation of the phenomenon of interest.

## HUMAN DRUG TRIAL GONE WRONG?

This is no doubt verging into the exclusive territory of conspiracy theorists. Nonetheless, it remains an alternative and plausible explanation of the outbreak given that there is no credible information on the existence of a likely Patient Zero, as well as no explanation of how the Zaire Ebola virus emerged in the middle of West Africa, about two thousand miles away from where it normally resides.

Three years before the 2014 outbreak in parts of West Africa, *The Guardian* (July 04, 2011) reported that the number of clinical trials in developing countries had surged to the extent that, by 2008, it was estimated that there were about three times as many developing countries participating in clinical trials registered with the United States Food and Drug Administration (USFDA) than there were in the whole period between 1948 and 2000. It noted further that pharmaceutical companies are attracted by the lower costs and availability of "treatment-naïve" patients, who are less likely to have been previously exposed to trials or similar drugs. On the other hand, developing countries are wooed by the promise of advanced medical technology and access to the latest and most effective treatments. Nonetheless, the governments of most African countries seldom set up a comprehensive and viable legal and ethical framework to protect their citizens participating in these trials. There is hardly ever any single international standard of ethical research to which foreign companies are expected to adhere, and hardly any national standard of ethical research to start with. Thus, corrupt politicians and immoral researchers are ardent bedfellows that may have easily teamed up as the fiendish angels of death by the Ebola virus.

On the 10<sup>th</sup> of March 2014, Michael Carome published an article in *The Huffington Post* intimating that unethical clinical trials are still being conducted in developing countries. He talked about the clinical trials that involved testing new methods of preventing the spread of HIV infection from mother to child that was reported by the Public Citizen's Health Research Group. The researchers had randomly assigned some pregnant women infected with the virus to receive placebos or other medications known to be ineffective. These wide-eyed women were certainly used as a test group, implying that they did not receive any active medication; their pain and slow death being factors that helped the researchers to determine whether the other group that received active medication was being treated by the medication. Michael Carome equally talked about the trial conducted in India to test the effectiveness of two rotavirus vaccines. This involved giving placebo injections of salt water rather than the vaccines to more than 2000 Indian children.

The Center for Research on Multinational Corporations published a paper in 2008 providing a more vivid picture of the problem. The paper discussed many examples of unethical human clinical trials in the 1990s and 2000s. In 1996, following the outbreak of meningitis in Kano, Nigeria, a trial of Trovafloxacin, a new quinolone antibiotic, was performed on children without obtaining the consent of their parents. The latter were simply unaware of the fact that their children were being experimented upon. Moreover, the Health Research Ethics Committee of Nigeria did not approve of the trial or so it claimed after the fact. Five of the children enrolled in the trial died, while others suffered paralysis and brain damage.

Between 1997 and 2003, Ugandan women who had been given the anti-transmission drug, Nevirapine, experienced several serious adverse effects. 14 of them died. Some of them were administered wrong doses; their consent was not obtained about changes in the experiment, and their symptoms were not reported.

In 2003, the drug streptokinase that was designed to treat clot-bursting in heart attacks and diabetes was tested on unwitting patients and without the permission of the Genetic Engineering Approval Committee. Eight of the patients died.

In the same year, the VGV-1 drug, an anti-HIV preparation was administered to HIV-positive patients in China without informing them of the adverse effects. They were not informed of the results of the trials.

Between 2004 and 2005, about 400 sex workers in Cameroon participated in a trial of the drug, Tenofovir, which was designed to prevent HIV transmission. However, their consent was not obtained since they were not properly informed about the risks. In fact, information was only provided in English, although most of the participants were French-speaking. At least five of the women were reported to have become HIV-infected while they were enrolled in the study. The trials were canceled in March 2005, one year before a similar trial was canceled in Cambodia. Interestingly, there is a strong possibility that each of the newly infected sex workers may have caused an outbreak in their respective villages or towns.

These are some of the examples of trials involving unwitting patients (usually poor and illiterate) in developing countries reported by the Center for Research on Multinational Corporations. It is only one of many reports of unethical trials conducted in developing countries. One of the most disconcerting cases not included in the report is that of the azidothymidine (AZT) trials that involved over 17,000 patients in Zimbabwe in the 1990s. This is well documented by Meier in an article published in *The Berkeley Journal of International Law* in 2002. The trials involved reputed researchers from the United States and were funded in part by the WHO, CDC, and the NIH. The consent of the patients was not obtained given that the testing methods and risks were not explained to them, as well as the nature of a placebo in clinical trials. Half of the "participants" received a placebo which made transmission of HIV to their fetuses likely. Thus, more than 1000 babies were allowed to be infected with the virus, although there were already established regimens that would have prevented this catastrophe. Interestingly, the trials were discontinued not because of a sudden pricking of the conscience but because the CDC believed it had already obtained enough information about the drug from trials conducted in Thailand.

This shows that there are many enlightened medicine men and women who have no qualms whatsoever about deliberately infecting other human beings, administering placebos to them after comforting and lying to them about the nature of the drug that has been injected into their systems, and observing them wilt and die over a given period. In the eyes of the researcher, there is no difference between the patient and a non-human primate (NHP) or guinea pig; maybe just slightly higher in the pecking order given that drugs such as AZT and Tenofovir were initially tested in macaques. With the gross lack of moral scruple and such strong malice aforethought, it is reasonable sometimes to presume human testing when many poor and illiterate people suddenly die from an infection, and subsequent researchers are unable to trace the source. As such, the contaminated needle that caused the outbreak of the Ebola virus disease may very well have been deliberately contaminated in order to infect unwitting "participants" in a clinical trial. Many drug trials with NHPs had already been conducted, and for the miscreant researcher, the next step would be trials with poor and illiterate humans, most likely in developing countries.

The unsavory background of unethical human clinical trials in developing countries often motivates mistrust as regards official statements about the causes of outbreaks and epidemics. This is especially the case where there are so many uncertainties and unanswered questions such as those concerning the 2014 outbreak of the Ebola virus disease in parts of West Africa. One of the most critical sets of questions in this regard concerns the sudden death of a prominent physician and his colleagues. The next chapter examines the questions.

# CHAPTER 6

# The Medicine Man of Kenema

It is noted in Chapter 1 that the Kenema Government Hospital is the reference hospital for hemorrhagic fever not only in the Eastern Province of Sierra Leone but also in the neighboring regions of Guinea and Liberia. It has the best stock of drugs for treating the symptoms of viral hemorrhagic fever such as severe diarrhea, kidney failure, and internal bleeding. It also has an isolation ward, the Lassa Fever Ward. Also, prior to the 2014 outbreak, many hemorrhagic fever experts from around the world worked at or with the Lassa Fever Ward. However, the laboratory at the ward is a Biosafety Level 2 laboratory, which is not equipped to deal with dangerous and virulent Biosafety Level 4 agents such as the Ebola virus. As such, following the outbreak of the Ebola virus disease in the region, the then Director, Sheikh Umar Khan, and other personnel at the ward knew that when a patient infected with the Ebola virus walked into the ward, they would be at a serious disadvantage. It was even more troubling that both Lassa and Ebola fevers may cause similar flulike symptoms such as cough, fever, general malaise, headache, and sore throat within the first day or days of infection. Thus, it must have been very confusing for the health personnel when a patient showing these systems began bleeding or had seizures or went into a coma. It could have been Lassa fever which is endemic in the region or the Ebola virus disease. Wynne Parry, in an article published on the *LiveScience* website dated November 08, 2012, shows how these diseases can be easily confused due to having similar symptoms. She cited Pardis Sabeti and Stephen Gire of Harvard University (and The Consortium) to the effect that the symptoms associated with Lassa and Ebola fevers may sometimes obscure their mundane manifestations. Both Pardis Sabeti and Stephen Gire conducted research on Lassa fever at the Kenema Government Hospital in Sierra Leone and Irrua Specialist Teaching Hospital in Nigeria. They also compared the manifestation of the Lassa fever to that of the Ebola fever.

Although it is understandable that any health personnel may have confused Lassa fever with Ebola fever, it is surprising that the experienced staff using personal protective equipment (PPE) at the Kenema Government Hospital did not take appropriate steps to isolate all the patients suspected to be suffering from any of the viral hemorrhagic fevers. This is especially the case with the patients that showed more serious symptoms such as hemorrhaging in the eyes, nose, or gums, repeated vomiting, respiratory distress, pain in the abdomen, and facial swelling. The CDC states that 20% of patients suffering from a viral hemorrhagic fever show these serious symptoms, and a third of the patients suffer from hearing loss. Also, the fact that the Lassa fever is endemic in Sierra Leone implies that the staff would have had to employ the requisite preventive measures many times in the past. Thus, they knew that the virus that causes hemorrhagic fever may be transmitted from one person to another after exposure to the virus in the tissue, blood, secretions or excretions of the patient. Also, they knew fully well that nosocomial transmission is high where the health personnel does not use PPE. In fact, there is no doubt about the latter point given that the former chief physician of the Lassa Fever Research Program at the Kenema Government Hospital, Aniru

Conteh, was infected by a contaminated needle stick and died from Lassa fever in 2004.

As such, the preventive measures taken to isolate patients suspected of having Lassa fever, until the disease ran its course, would have equally prevented the spread of the Ebola virus disease within the hospital. Experienced staff who had dealt with several cases of Lassa virus infection in the past would have taken these recommended barrier nursing methods and worn protective clothing including gloves, masks, gowns, and goggles. They would also have sterilized their equipment. The Consortium claimed that the Lassa Fever Ward of the Kenema General Hospital, although a dingy cabin, was very well equipped. It is, therefore, surprising that the healthcare personnel of the ward were quickly infected by the Ebola virus, only a few months after the outbreak. Given their experience in dealing with Lassa fever that is endemic in the region, and also the fact that there was no reported case of Ebola in the region prior to the outbreak, it may be surmised that patients that showed symptoms of a hemorrhagic fever would have been thought to have been infected with the Lassa virus. In this instance, the health personnel would have used the recommended preventive measures to prevent transmission from person to person. As noted above, these preventive measures would equally have been effective in preventing the transmission of the Ebola virus that these patients carried to the health personnel and other persons. This is because the Ebola virus may only spread through direct contact with a patient's broken skin, mucous membranes, blood and other body fluids, and contaminated objects (such as needles and syringes). Hence, the isolation precaution or preventive measures recommended to prevent the spread of the Lassa fever would have been effective in containing the Ebola virus within the Lassa Fever Ward of the hospital.

The question that follows is why this was not the case. It was later on reported that the hospital was simply inundated with the growing number of patients and the overwhelmed healthcare workers soon found themselves in the virus' line of fire given that they could not handle the flock with their overstretched and under-resourced service. Statistics from the Ministry of Health and Sanitation of Sierra Leone show that the Kenema Government Hospital received 504 patients suffering from the Ebola virus disease. 307 of them were subsequently discharged, and 197 died. It is difficult to imagine how the small dingy cabins and makeshift structures would have contained 504 patients suffering from the Ebola virus disease, as well as an even larger number of patients suffering from many other diseases. Hence, at the time the hospital looked like a congested clinic in a bombed monastery in a war-ravaged city. There is certainly no doubt that the healthcare workers were stretched too thin. And so scores of them (doctors, nurses, and support staff) died from the Ebola virus disease. Amongst this group of true heroes were two of the most experienced and beloved members of the Lassa Fever Ward personnel, the director, Sheikh Umar Khan, and the chief nurse, Mbalu Fonnie. This chapter seeks to understand why the workers at the Lassa Fever Ward (the senior providers especially) could not be saved despite the fact they had a close relationship with many viral hemorrhagic fever experts around the world. It attempts to determine whether they simply voluntarily suffered death as the penalty for witnessing the devastating spread of the Ebola virus disease in Kenema.

## DEATH OF THE MEDICINE MAN

A glowing tribute is paid to Sheikh Umar Khan in the *Antiviral Research* journal of November 2014. He was born in 1975 in Lungi, a coastal town in Port Loko in the Northern Province of Sierra Leone. The sea separates Lungi from the nation's capital, Freetown. Khan was the youngest of 10 children and proudly referred to himself as "doctor" as a young child. That became reality when he graduated from the College of Medicine and Allied Health Sciences of the

University of Sierra Leone in 2001. He then completed his internship three years later. In 2005, he became the chief physician of the Lassa Fever Research Program at the Kenema Government Hospital following the death of Aniru Conteh, who previously held the post. As mentioned above, the latter died from Lassa fever after being infected by a contaminated needle stick. Thus, Sheikh Umar Khan had a good grasp of the risk of working on the Lassa fever program at Kenema before taking up office. For him, that entailed moving to the hinterlands, which is an ordeal for the educated African. This more than anything demonstrates that the young physician was prepared to endure great suffering in order to uphold a principle or further a cause. He directed patient care at the Lassa Fever Ward and carried out in-depth studies on Lassa fever and other diseases as evidenced by several publications that he co-authored. Prominent amongst these are publications in the *Antiviral Research* journal, *Clinical Infectious Diseases* journal, *PLOS Neglected Tropical Diseases* journal, and the *Emerging Infectious Diseases* journal.

Between 2010 and 2013, he underwent specialist training in internal medicine at the West African College of Physicians in Accra, Ghana. While at this college, he came close to being infected by HIV. He was pierced by an infected needle stick while drawing blood from a patient with AIDS. He prevented infection by implementing post-exposure chemoprophylaxis promptly. This involves taking two to three antiretroviral medications immediately after possible exposure to HIV (before the virus has had time to make too many copies of itself in the person's body) in order to minimize the chances of becoming HIV positive. Khan soon returned to Sierra Leone but did not take up a more lucrative position in the city. The tribute article in the *Antiviral Research* journal notes that he was keen on re-joining the clinical and research team in Kenema. That decision proved costly. His time of tribulation began as soon as the following year. The sudden and unexpected occurrence of the Ebola virus disease hit

Kenema especially hard. This may be due to the fact that the Kenema Government Hospital is a highly regarded medical center in the region and received the most complex cases since it had better machinery and equipment. As chief physician of the Lassa Fever Research Program and given his experience and training, he was no doubt the local viral hemorrhagic fever expert and logically saw patients and coordinated the valiant efforts of a flustered and disconcerted personnel that almost always relied on resources that had been stretched thin. The tribute article in the *Antiviral Research* journal paints the picture of a physician who had voluntarily put himself through anguish as a penalty for staying the course and helping out. His sister, Aissata, is quoted to have admonished him against working at the makeshift Ebola treatment center, to which he had retorted "I am afraid for my life, I must say … Health workers are prone to the disease because we are the first port of call for somebody who is sickened by disease." But then he noted that "If I refuse to treat them, who would treat me?"

An article by Andrew Pollack published in *The New York Times* (August 12, 2014) described the ordeal of Sheikh Umar Khan's last days. He tested positive for Ebola on July 21, 2014, and died eight days later. While he lay dying from the Ebola virus disease, his international colleagues faced the dilemma of administering the drug, ZMAPP or hope he could be recover like 45% of patients who survived without treatment. Andrew Pollack noted that they were in a quandary because the drug had never before been tested on people. Thus, it was uncertain whether the drug would help or instead kill the physician faster. In the latter instance, public trust in international organizations would have been shattered as many Africans, already suspicious of these organizations, would have accused them of testing their drug on the African physician. Armand Sprecher from *Médecins Sans Frontières* is quoted as saying that they feared killing Sheikh Umar Khan with the drug. He also said Sheikh Umar Khan's virus levels were already so high that they believed the drug would probably not have worked in any event. Andrew Pollack also stated that Sheikh Umar Khan has since been moved from the Lassa Fever Ward in Kenema to the medical center set up by *Médecins Sans Frontières* in Kailahun so that he would not be treated by his colleagues. Moreover, his treatment team planned on airlifting him to Switzerland, but the transportation company refused to take him because he was already vomiting and suffering from diarrhea.

It is, however, surprising that the question whether to administer the experimental drug, ZMAPP, to Sheikh Umar Khan was raised by his treatment team only when his virus levels were already too high. They had ample time to consider this in the early days of the infection but did not. Also, they did not seek his opinion as regards whether he would volunteer to take the drug. Given that the drug had undergone successful clinical trials on NHPs, it was not exactly a case of choosing between the devil and the deep blue sea. Daniel Bausch, who was among the writers of the tribute article in the *Antiviral Research* journal, is cited by Andrew Pollack (*The New York Times*) as disagreeing with the decision not to administer ZMAPP to Sheikh Umar Khan. Daniel Bausch said if he had a terminal disease he would certainly have preferred to take his chances with a drug that had not undergone safety testing. He also deplored the fact that the treatment team did not seek Sheikh Umar Khan's opinion, which was a very informed opinion. From Daniel Bausch's statement, it is clear that if Sheikh Umar Khan had not been moved to Kailahun, his colleagues at the Lassa Fever Ward would have sought to obtain and administer the drug to him.

Interestingly, ZMAPP was administered to two American aid workers who became infected. They were then airlifted to Emory University Hospital in Atlanta. They both survived. Spanish authorities secured the drug for a Spanish priest who had also been infected in Liberia, but he died from the disease. Nonetheless, the treatment team in Madrid refused to confirm whether they had administered the drug to the ailing priest. It is also surprising that no attempt was made to use TKM-Ebola which had been tested in a human clinical trial as shown above. A prominent partner of The Consortium, Thomas Geisbert, had worked on the development of TKM-Ebola. Thus, Sheikh Umar Khan had acquaintances (at The Consortium) who had access to experimental drugs that had gone through clinical trials, yet, no attempt was made to administer any of the drugs to him. As regards TKM-Ebola, although Phase II of the human clinical trial conducted during the crisis showed that the drug is not effective, it is surprising that a desperate attempt was not made to test the drug on the medicine man of Kenema. This is because the drug was subsequently tested on other patients during the Phase II clinical trial conducted during the crisis.

As regards ZMAPP, an article by Qiu et al. published in the *Scientific Reports* journal on November 28, 2013, noted that non-human primates that were dosed with ZMab within 24 or 48 hours after exposure demonstrated robust immune responses to the Ebola virus. They were rechallenged 10 or 13 weeks after the first challenge with another dose of ZMab. This drug was created by Defyrus, a company that develops military measures to restore biosecurity. It is a blend of three antibodies including mAbs: m1H3, m2G4, and m4G7. Qiu et al. in a paper published in the *Nature* journal in August 2014 describe how these three antibodies were chimerized and then tested in guinea pigs and NHPs with combinations of MB-003 in order to determine the best combination. The latter was then termed ZMapp. The paper notes further that 21 rhesus macaque monkeys were infected with the Congolese Kikwit variant of the Zaire Ebola virus. These monkeys are native to South, Central, and Southeast Asia and share approximately 93% of DNA sequence with humans. They may also have had a common ancestor some 25 million years ago. The Kikwit variant is that which caused the outbreak in the Democratic Republic of Congo (Zaire) in early 1995. Some of the infected primates received three doses of ZMapp. They survived, while the other primates died. A paper by Thomas Geisbert also published in the *Nature* journal in August 2014 noted that ZMapp had prevented the replication of the Makon variant of the Zaire Ebola virus. The latter variant caused the 2014 outbreak in parts of West Africa. The findings reported by Qiu et al. before this outbreak (*Scientific Reports*, November 28, 2013) show that ZMapp had the potential to treat primates if administered shortly after infection. It had effectively treated rhesus macaque monkeys that share about 93% of DNA sequence with humans. Equally, as noted above, TKM-Ebola that had already been used in a human clinical trial (Phase I), although the results have neither been discussed nor published. Notwithstanding, what is important is that the papers by Qiu et al. and Thomas Geisbert show that the decision to administer ZMapp to Sheikh Umar Khan was not the same as the decision to offer a totally unproven drug to an unwitting patient. It was already established that this drug had a strong potential as regards treating Ebola patients. That explains why there were no qualms about administering the drug to the American and European healthcare workers who became infected during the crisis.

It is therefore still difficult to understand why Sheikh Umar Khan was left to die. Shortly after the experimental drugs were administered to two American healthcare workers and allegedly to a Spanish priest, a panel set up by the WHO comprising researchers, regulators, and ethicists said it was ethical to offer experimental drugs to treat or prevent the spread of the Ebola virus. Alta Charo, Professor of Law and Bioethics at the University of Wisconsin is cited by Susan Brink in a blog on NPR's website (12 August 2014) as stating that the biggest moral quandary posed by a rapidly spreading disease and very limited supply of (unproven) drugs is who gets the drug first. It is argued that in a public health crisis, it is reasonable to offer the drug to the people who can save other people first. Thus, priority must be given to healthcare personnel and other first responders because they must be kept alive. This certainly justifies administering the experimental drug to the American and European healthcare workers. However, one of the most prominent Sierra Leonean healthcare workers who was ironically hailed as the face of the country's fight against Ebola was not given this privilege.

Susan Brink noted that under American law, the FDA may permit a manufacturer to provide an experimental drug to patients where there are no alternatives and the consequences of doing nothing are severe. She discussed the example of Anthony Fauci, the then Director of the National Institute of Allergy and Infectious Diseases, who allowed the growing number of AIDS patients access to the unapproved AZT outside of clinical trials. However, she stated that these exceptions are often granted when the drug is in a clinical trial, and unlike the AZT, the drugs for the Ebola virus disease were not yet in human clinical trials. The latter statement is incorrect given that TKM-Ebola was already in a human clinical trial prior to the outbreak of the Ebola virus disease in West Africa. The FDA put the trial on hold in the middle of July 2014 in order to effectively assess the effects of the drug. That was about seven months after the outbreak. Notwithstanding, the argument here is that there was a strong moral case to offer the experimental drugs to the infected healthcare workers, and the decision to let Sheikh Umar Khan die is therefore highly exceptionable. There was outrage at the fact that the drugs were offered to American and European healthcare workers but not to African healthcare workers. The outrage is justified to the extent that African healthcare workers as important as Sheikh Umar Khan were not given this lifeline.

Salim S. Abdool Karim, the Director of an AIDS research center in South Africa is cited by *The New York Times* (article by Andrew Pollack, August 08, 2014) to the effect that if the experimental drugs had been administered to Africans first, "it would have been front-page screaming headline: Africans used as guinea pigs for American drug company's medicine." This argument is not only slightly stupid and disingenuous but also a mark of disrespect to the departed African healthcare workers who could have been saved by the experimental drugs. As an African, Salim S. Abdool Karim knows only too well that suspicion and indignation characterize the attitude of many Africans (especially rural and poorly educated urban dwellers) toward Western medicine men. This is in part a vestige of colonialism and in part due to the fact that many African countries have so many times been the sites of many unethical clinical trials over the centuries (some examples are discussed in Chapter 5). Harriet Washington provides a good justification for this attitude in an article in *The New York Times* published on July 31, 2007, and a book, *Medical Apartheid: The Dark History of Medical Experimentation on Black Americans from Colonial Times to the Present.* As such, it is hard to argue that the risk of public outrage in Africa would deter Western medicine men from administering a drug in good faith to dying patients in a medical emergency. In fact, given the cynicism with which the outcry by Africans is often received, an impassioned uproar would almost always be interpreted as crying wolf. Moreover, dealing with healthcare workers is very different from dealing with subjects that do not understand the possible dangers or the nature of the drug. It was, therefore, important to seek Sheikh Umar Khan's opinion, especially given his knowledge of the disease and supposed knowledge of the research on treatment therapies. Also, neither the WHO nor Kentucky BioProcessing (Reynolds American) were going to announce that they had administered the experimental drug to the African healthcare workers immediately after the event. Such information usually becomes public several months and sometimes years after the event.

The management of Sheikh Umar Khan's case may be contrasted with the management of the cases of the virologists' accidental exposure to the Ebola virus in the Bernhard Nocht Institute's laboratory in Germany and USAMRIID's Biosafety Level 4 laboratory. These cases are discussed in Chapter 5. As regards the exposure in Germany, a teleconference was held on the same day with researchers in the United States and Canada to discuss potential treatments. After the teleconference, a vaccine known as the VSVΔG/ZEBOVGP was shipped to Hamburg, Germany from Winnipeg, Canada; and an emergency clearance from customs was obtained. The following day, another teleconference was held with several filovirus researchers from American and Canadian institutions, including the USAMRIID and the University of Texas Medical Branch. The VSVΔG/ZEBOVGP vaccine was administered to the virologist two days after exposure. This was in 2009, some five years before the outbreak of the Ebola virus disease in parts of West Africa. The exposure in the United States was even earlier, in 2004. They considered administering the untested recombinant nematode protein (rNAPc2) and antisense oligomers if the virologist who had been exposed showed evidence of infection. Thus, it is disingenuous and almost condescending to contend that the risk of public outrage or uncertainty about the effects of the experimental drugs deterred the physicians taking care of Sheikh Umar Khan from administering the drugs to him. This was in 2014, ten years after the case in the United States. Although a conspiracy to let the medicine man of Kenema join the heavenly choir may be far-fetched, it is likely that these physicians knew that the available stock of experimental drugs was quite limited; and that since the disease was still wreaking havoc, many American and European healthcare workers would be infected. Hence, it was more of a question of the controlled distribution of scarce resources. If they had successfully treated Sheikh Umar Khan with the experimental drug, they would have been overwhelmed by demand for the drug from other African healthcare workers.

As such, what is most disheartening and outrageous in this story is that Sheikh Umar Khan is not the only West African healthcare provider and frontline worker who was left to die, even though the experimental drugs were available. Four other healthcare workers who equally worked at the Lassa Fever Ward got infected and died. They include the mother figure of the staff, Mbalu Fonnie, who had worked as nurse and midwife at the Kenema Government Hospital for more than 30 years; Mohammed Fullah, a laboratory technician at the Lassa Fever Ward; and Alex Moigboi and Alice Kovoma, both nurses at the ward. It is quite strange that these workers at the Lassa Fever Ward were allegedly conducting a study on the causes of the outbreak, but all suddenly died before their findings were ever published. Even more alarming is that a sixth co-author, Sidiki Safa, who worked on the same study and was not infected, suddenly died from a stroke before the findings were submitted and published.

The subsequent publication of the work revealed that they were allegedly involved in a study with maybe 44 other researchers. They were sequencing the genomes of samples taken from 78 infected patients (totaling 99 viral genomes) in order to determine how the virus spread. However, the findings of the study were only submitted to the *Science* journal on August 05, 2014, after all the researchers at the Lassa Fever Ward had passed. The paper was published on August 21, 2014. Some of the surviving co-authors are researchers that are cited in this book, including Stephen Gire, Pardis Sabeti, and Robert F. Garry, prominent members of The Consortium. Some of the findings of the study as reported in the article in the *Science* journal are somewhat controversial. It is for example submitted that there was indeed a natural reservoir, although no evidence is adduced to this effect. It is difficult to understand why the article notes that continued human-reservoir exposure was unlikely to have contributed to the growth of the epidemic, and yet maintains that there was a natural reservoir. What natural reservoir would infect one human and then vanish without a trace, and without transmitting the virus to other animals or humans? Notwithstanding, what is most controversial about this paper is that many of the healthcare workers who did the groundwork died from the Ebola virus disease although they could have been saved.

# A Flurry of Questions

The host-seeking behavior of viruses is well-established. However, researchers are still unable to tell why some viruses like the Ebola virus seem to appear out of nowhere and disappear into thin air after an uproar. Despite categorical media statements and the posturing of some pompous researchers, there is still no evidence that humans have disturbed the natural reservoir of the Ebola virus by hunting it for meat or dragging it out of its ecosystem. This shows that unless it is the researcher that causes the virus to venture out into a new host, the researcher's postulate about the spillover event and outbreak would largely be based on speculation. All the spillover events since 1976 have so far gone unnoticed as many animal and human hosts provide a dead end for the transmission of the Ebola virus disease. Thus, given that the natural reservoir remains unknown, the spillover event has become the upshot of speculation. But then again, why do researchers continue to talk of a 'natural' reservoir? One would no doubt be hard-pressed to find any article in a peer-reviewed journal that casts doubt on the fact that the Ebola virus disease is a zoonotic disease. It has also been established that each of the last three previous outbreaks of the Ebola virus disease in Africa represents an independent zoonotic event from the same genetically diverse viral population in its natural reservoir. However, this does not necessarily imply that the outbreak in 2014 in parts of West Africa began with a single zoonotic transmission event, but that the Ebola virus responsible for the outbreak came from Central or Middle Africa (where there had been a zoonotic transmission event) sometime between 2004 and 2014. Researchers ransacked the West African forest and found no evidence of any decline in the population of remaining large mammals in the area, but ironically, they found evidence of the increase in the population of chimpanzees. Thus, it is uncertain what animal or natural reservoir would infect one or few humans and then vanish without a trace and without transmitting the virus to other animals or humans. One may go out on a limb and surmise that the natural reservoirs may be humans given that the Ebola virus may live in some humans (who have antibodies against the virus) in a suppressed state, and may re-emerge when their immune systems collapse. Nonetheless, if this nonviable surmission were true, the human reservoirs would continue to feed the outbreak with new transmissions.

As such, in an attempt to address the many questions that have beset many objective observers following the outbreak of the Ebola virus disease in parts of West Africa, it is argued here that the claim about a non-animal source is not altogether extraordinary. There is consensus on the fact that the outbreak stemmed from *a single transmission of the virus to the index case*, without further exposure of any humans to the source. This implies that after the first transmission of the virus from the source, no other human came in contact with that source. Also, one of the most prominent researchers, Sylvain Baize, is cited by Denise Grady and Sheri Fink in *The New York Times* as stating that the outbreak may have been caused by a contaminated fruit or "An injection with a contaminated needle." It is shown above that despite the most rigorous of safety measures in Biosafety Level 4 laboratories in Germany, the United States, and Russia, there have been documented laboratory accidents with the Ebola virus. Hence, an accident in a laboratory causing the outbreak is a strong theoretical possibility. Also, the American media and some American researchers have accused the Russians of seeking to weaponize the Ebola virus, while the latter have also accused American researchers of equally trying to weaponize the pathogen. There is no evidence to support any of the accusations. However, what is certain is that in both countries, researchers have used man-made variants of the Ebola virus in conducting bioterrorism research in laboratories owned or managed by the military.

Nonetheless, what is important to note is that if research on the Ebola virus is fraught with peril in enclosed laboratory facilities that are designed for work with very dangerous and exotic pathogens, one can only imagine how far more dangerous it is to work with the Ebola virus in a laboratory that is not suited for such work. It is extremely dangerous to work with the virus in a laboratory with a low level of containment designed for work with agents of only moderate potential hazard. Thus, if the virus had, for example, arrived in deep-frozen blood samples at the Biosafety Level 2 laboratory of the Lassa Fever Ward of the Kenema Government Hospital in Sierra Leone, any study conducted on the virus there would have increased the risk of exposure to exponential levels. This scenario is not altogether far-fetched given that studies on the Ebola virus disease were conducted by some prominent members of the partnership of research institutes (The Consortium) that seeks to promote health and safety around the world by creating new diagnostic procedures and therapies and reducing the incidence of viral hemorrhagic fevers. It is shown above that the company, Autoimmune Technologies, and the prominent researcher, Thomas Geisbert (Texas University) conducted extensive studies on the Ebola virus disease prior to the 2014 outbreak. Tulane University (also part of The Consortium) has noted that it effectively conducted biodefense-related studies at the Kenema Government

Hospital between 2010 and 2014. Also, it has insinuated that the interest of the National Institute of Allergy and Infectious Diseases (NIAID) of the NIH in The Consortium's research project (and the motivation for awarding $15 million) was related to the fact that the Lassa virus is a Biosafety Level 4 (BSL-4) and NIAID Biodefense category A agent that may potentially be used as a biological weapon directed against civilian or military targets. As such, it may be assumed that the NIAID sought to ensure that Tulane University (and The Consortium) developed counter-threat measures such as vaccines, therapeutics, and diagnostic assays. Beyond the obvious question of why Ebola virus disease experts were involved with The Consortium when the latter has repeatedly claimed that its research prior to the outbreak was exclusively focused on the Lassa virus, one cannot help but be curious about The Consortium's strange focus on the "bioterrorism threats" posed by the Ebola and Lassa viruses, despite the fact that there is no evidence of the existence of any forms of the viruses adapted for use as weapons of war. Did this simply constitute a subterfuge to ensure that partners of The Consortium obtain funding from the government of the United States?

In August 2014, the government of the United States decided not to renew funding for the research project on Lassa fever and thereby cut resources for the Lassa Fever Ward of the Kenema Government Hospital. At the time the ward had more or less become the Ebola ward, given that it was used to treat the large numbers of patients who had contracted the lethal Ebola virus disease. A contracting officer for NIAID intimated that the proposal for the renewal of funding submitted by Tulane University had been rejected "based on technical factors, scientific priority, and availability of funds." The NIH declined to provide any clarifications or even comment further. The timing of the decision and the uncertainty as regards the NIH's motivation certainly raise many questions. Was the decision related to the government's decision to cut spending? Does the uncommunicative posture imply the NIH had caught a whiff of something unethical cooking in Kenema prior to the outbreak?

On July 23, 2014, the Sierra Leonean Ministry of Health and Sanitation ordered Tulane University "to stop Ebola testing during the current Ebola outbreak." It is uncertain whether this implies that the Ministry had sanctioned research on Ebola by Tulane University prior to the outbreak, and it was advising the latter to cease "Ebola testing" during the outbreak. For starters, what is "Ebola testing" and why did the Sierra Leonean government suddenly become apprehensive?

On June 19, 2015, Tekmira released a press statement to the effect that the Phase II of the human clinical trial of TKM-Ebola-Guinea had reached a predefined statistical endpoint and enrolment had been closed. This implies that the experimental drug, an anti-Ebola RNAi therapeutic that targets the Zaire Ebola virus (Makona variant), did not work on patients in Sierra Leone and "was not likely to demonstrate an overall therapeutic benefit" if enrolment continued. However, the chief investigator, Peter Horby, intimated that the order by the Sierra Leonean Ministry of Health and Sanitation to Tulane University (The Consortium) to "stop Ebola testing" was not one of the reasons that motivated the decision to discontinue the human clinical trial. It was stopped because of meeting a pre-defined statistical endpoint. But then he said he had no information about the results of the Phase I trial. This is quite strange since conducting the Phase II trial surely implies that the experimental drug had been deemed relatively safe following the results of the Phase I trial. In other words, the findings of the Phase I trial ought to have justified the carrying out of Phase II, given that if the drugs were neither effective nor safe following administration to a small group of humans during Phase I, it would have been unethical to proceed with Phase II whereby the drug was administered to a larger group of humans. Thus, it is important to determine the results of the Phase I trial and also confirm where the trial was conducted and who were the healthy volunteers used. What is most disturbing here is that the Phase I trial was conducted in an undisclosed location, using undisclosed healthy volunteers, and *prior to* the outbreak of the Ebola virus disease in parts of West Africa. The non-disclosure of the results, as well as the fact that the chief investigator of the Phase II trial is unaware of the results, are frankly speaking very troubling.

It follows from the above that since Guinea, Liberia, and Sierra Leone were not considered areas in which the Zaire Ebola virus was present prior to 2014, and there were Ebola virus disease experts in Sierra Leone conducting studies on Ebola (and other hemorrhagic fevers) shortly before the outbreak, then the likelihood that the outbreak may have been caused by a laboratory accident or clinical trial that went wrong, is fairly high. This is only logical given that a laboratory accident or clinical trial is the nearest cause in the chain or network of possible causes of the outbreak. The other causes such as zoonotic transmission are more improbable in the postulated sequence of events given that there is no trace of the virus in any animal (whether potential natural reservoir or not) in the affected regions. However, there is no conclusive evidence that a laboratory accident or human clinical trial is the preponderant cause. No researcher or Institute (including those of The Consortium) has admitted in public that it conducted human clinical trials in Sierra Leone or Guinea prior to the 2014 outbreak, or worse that there was an accidental exposure to the Ebola virus. The Consortium has always maintained that the studies of its partners were focused on Lassa fever which is endemic in the region. Nonetheless, prominent researchers have in the past announced that they were studying one disease when in fact they were conducting a combined study (involving the Ebola virus). It is noted above that many reasons (mischief aside) may explain this strategy: lack of funding, lack of support from the hierarchy, sensitiveness of the study, etc. The example of members of the International Commission that was set up to combat the Ebola virus disease in Zaire in 1976 is discussed. They sought to identify the reservoir and any antibodies in the reservoir's blood after their mission to contain the disease in the Bumba area was complete. Unable to obtain funding to this effect, they submitted a proposal for funding their research on monkeypox and then conducted a combined study on both monkeypox and Ebola. They collected samples from 117 species in the Ebola hotspot; the animals were mostly trapped or hunted by the local villagers in exchange for monetary rewards offered by the researchers. However, the samples collected by these researchers were not handled in a Biosafety Level 4 laboratory, implying that the risk of exposure to the virus was extremely high. The researchers surely knew of the risk only so well but went ahead with the study. If the virus were then dragged out of its ecosystem, that would have caused another outbreak, and it is hard to believe that the researchers would have admitted in public that the outbreak was caused by exposure to the virus during a furtive study. The fault would no doubt have been imputed to the villagers who had an unquenchable appetite for game.

This takes us to the official narrative about the 2014 outbreak. It is shown above that a two-year-old child, Emile Ouamonou, has unfortunately become the protagonist of the Ebola tragedy because for some unspecified reason some oblivious researchers and many impulsive journalists have decided to identify him as the index case, rather than the point where the chains of transmission seemed to have ended as per the first epidemiologic study conducted shortly after the outbreak. Several researchers traveled to Guinea and Sierra Leone, captured bats and other animals and collected blood and tissue samples and found no evidence of a zoonotic transmission. Also, they have found no evidence of any decline in the population of remaining large mammals in the area. But strange enough, some of them continue to hold that a mysterious bat somehow made contact with the two-year-old alone in a hollow tree, 50 meters away from their home, and then did not infect any other animal or person in or around the village or region.

It is shown above that despite the fact that there is still a strong case for arguing that Emile Ouamonou and members of his family may have died from the Ebola virus disease, it remains that the contention that Emile is Patient Zero is tenuous. First, it is uncertain whether he was not infected by his mother or grandmother. The fact that he allegedly died before the latter does not necessarily imply that he transmitted the virus to them. The Ebola virus disease is most deadly among babies and toddlers. They get sick faster as the average incubation period is about seven days in babies, but could last for up to 21 days in adults. As such, it is more likely that Emile picked up the virus from his 25-year-old mother or 46-year-old grandmother but died first since the incubation period is much shorter for babies and toddlers. His four-year-old sister died shortly after him.

Secondly, Emile is least likely to have come into contact with the host or reservoir of the virus. Many studies have concluded that there was only a single introduction of the virus into the population due to the high degree of similarity among the gene sequences and the epidemiologic links between the cases. 'Single introduction' implies a chance encounter with the animal source (zoonotic transmission) or the ambitious researcher (nosocomial transmission). However, it is unlikely that a two-year-old in a crowded home would wander aimlessly into the woods, and he was already quite sick before his parents took him to the local clinic. Also, Baize et al. believe that the introduction may have happened in December 2013. However, if Emile died on the 06th of December, then the introduction happened in November. But if he died on the 28th of December (*Zeit Online*), then he certainly was not the index case as the incubation period for toddlers is seven to ten days. As noted above, the fact that his grandmother died on the 1st of January 2014 implies that she got infected sometime around the first week of December. Equally, the fact that Emile died on the 28th of December implies that he got infected sometime around the 19th or 20th of December. As such, the odd insistence on identifying Emile as the index case despite all evidence to the contrary only feeds the suspicion of dishonest behavior at the onset of the crisis.

Nonetheless, the strong suspicion of unlawful or dishonest behavior resulting in the outbreak of the Ebola virus disease cannot be dissociated from the fact that the story has largely been told from a non-African perspective. As noted in Chapter 2, information about the outbreak of the disease in Africa was received with mixed feelings in different parts of the world. For many in Europe, Asia, and North America, it was the obvious and hackneyed sarcastic retort about those Africans who have infected themselves by eating monkeys and bats. However, for many in Africa (and other poor parts of the world), it was the obvious and overdone glorification of the state of being a victim: the result of another illegal medical experimentation by those White people. After all, in 1996, following the outbreak of meningitis in Kano, Nigeria, a trial of Trovafloxacin was performed on children without obtaining the consent of their parents. Five of the children died. Between 1997 and 2003, unwitting Ugandan women who had been given the anti-transmission drug, Nevirapine, experienced several serious adverse effects. 14 of them died. Between 2004 and 2005, about 400 unwitting sex workers in Cameroon participated in a trial of the drug, Tenofovir, which was designed to prevent HIV transmission. At least five of the women were reported to have become HIV-infected while they were enrolled in the study. During AZT trials in Zimbabwe in the 1990s, thousands of "participants" received a placebo which made transmission of HIV to their fetuses likely. More than 1000 babies were allowed to be infected with the virus, although there were already established regimen that would have prevented this 'epidemic.' And these are only some of the reported unethical trials. The majority of such trials are obviously kept secret. Hence, the experience of victimization has logically resulted in the spread of fear and suspicion in the affected African community. On the other hand, there is a correspondence bias that explains the thwarted judgment by many non-Africans in more affluent societies. They are largely disposed toward focusing on dispositional or personality-based explanations for the observed behavior of Africans while overlooking situational explanations.

Notwithstanding, many bloggers or 'conspiracy theorists' are criticized above for making false analogies owing to the fact that they use the perceived similarities between the Flu virus and Ebola virus as the basis to infer some further similarity: outbreaks of diseases caused by both viruses are due to the experimentation on unsuspecting people. It was pointed out that the fact that both outbreaks are caused by viruses is not at all relevant to the question of whether Guinean or Sierra Leonean villagers were infected with the Ebola virus in order to test experimental drugs. Also, the fact that there is evidence of the modification of the Flu virus to one that may potentially infect humans is not at all relevant to the question of whether the variant of the Zaire Ebola virus that caused the outbreak in parts of West Africa is a laboratory-engineered variant that was somehow released from a US-funded research facility. It may equally be pointed out here that the fact that human clinical trials on unwitting Africans are ongoing is not at all relevant to the question of whether the 2014 outbreak of the Ebola virus disease was caused by a human clinical trial gone wrong. Despite a strong suspicion of foul play, it is an existential fallacy to presuppose that all disease pathogens (including the Ebola virus) have been modified (weaponized) and injected into unsuspecting Africans without evidence to this effect. Unfortunately, it is ironical that the only fact that has existential import here is the negligence and devil-may-care attitude of African authorities.

It is shown in Chapter 1 that while the rest of the world was panicky and hysterical, the epicenter of the Ebola virus disease was impassive and almost incautious. In fact news of the outbreak of the disease in Sierra Leone was greeted with skepticism by people who thought the news was politically motivated. The President of the Republic seemed to be engaging himself in more productive investments of his energy. His response was tardy and then followed by a most surreal appeal to the members of his cabinet and other officials involved in managing the crisis to stop embezzling funds allocated to this cause as that was "blood money." A report by the Auditor-General published on February 13, 2015, revealed that 30 percent of the US$19 million allegedly spent by the Sierra Leonean government in managing the crisis had been disbursed without proper supporting documentation. There was no evidence that incentive payments had been made to frontline healthcare workers, there were "ghost names" on some lists of healthcare workers, and some payments could not be accounted for. The Office of the President of the Republic then submitted the Auditor-General's report to Parliament rather than the police. This is not surprising, for health care and accountability have never been this country's top priorities. In fact, it epitomizes the paradox of poverty in modern Africa. It is among the top 15 diamond producing countries on the planet with a population of about 6 million, and yet boasts of one of the worst public health systems around the world.

The most depressing fact is the lack of interest in identifying the source of the outbreak and determining how the Zaire Ebola virus was able to travel thousands of miles away from the hot zone in Central or Middle Africa. What if the outbreak was caused by a bungled human clinical trial or an ambitious researcher who sneaked a frozen sample into the country? It may nonetheless be difficult for an African government to establish the truth because the vast majority of studies on the epidemiology and changes of the Ebola virus are published by American, European, and Asian researchers. It is noted above that the West African researchers who ought to have a much better understanding of the local culture and habits of the affected people are as scarce as the bones of antediluvian animals. Although the Western media (Western Europe and the United States) are only keen on hearing from African patients and families of patients, there is no reason why African governments should be as dismissive of their researchers. Very little is known of Sheikh Umar Khan's ideas and the research that he was conducting together with five other Sierra Leonean healthcare workers shortly before they all suddenly died. Everything about the physician and his ideas is found in articles published by European and American researchers. Apart from banners carrying his name and face, there is nothing to suggest that the Sierra Leoneans take much interest in the man. They are certainly owed an explanation as to why he was left to die. The decisions taken by the physicians attending to him were abysmally bizarre, to say the least, and may incite the locals to contend that the motive was sinister. It is also strange that neither the Kenema Government Hospital nor the ISTH of Nigeria contributes (at least intellectually) to the research on the effective ways of managing hemorrhagic fevers. There are no researchers from the ISTH working with The Consortium on the delineation of the mechanisms by which naturally occurring antibodies kill Ebola, Lassa, and Marburg viruses in order to ascertain vaccine designs and testing. The importance of these African structures is purely logistical. That may explain why things happen in Africa, and Africans turn to Europe and the United States and ask why.